Don't Blame McDonald's, Did Mommy Make You Fat?

Don Paullin
FatWarriorsNation.com

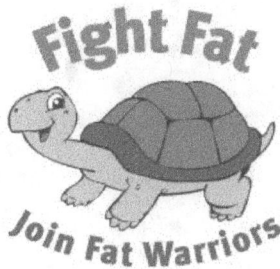

Fight Fat

Join Fat Warriors

ISBN: 978-0-9785314-2-3
Library of Congress Control Number: 2009921777

Printed in the United States of America
Publication Date: February 2009

Cover and interior property of Fat Warriors, Inc.
Cover design by Jason Shah
Interior book design and layout by Bookcovers.com

Business Certification Publishing, Inc.
Box 440
Grayslake, IL 60030

ACKNOWLEDGMENTS

I must thank all the profitable diet plans whose failures demanded I write this book. I especially was inspired by their quick and easy guarantees plus the bonus of before and after pictures. None of which I used for this book.

Beauty before age: Trish Boos who not only fought through the maze of my writing but inspired me to dig deeper. She worked her magic to help make my wandering writings into organized pages called a book. Thanks for being my weekend warrior editor.

Dick Juntunen has become my personal friend, loyal confidant and drill sergeant. Dick has tried to keep me moving like a writer should. He encouraged my creativity but kept me out of literary jail. This is the second book he has brought to production with me. Amazingly he is still somewhat sane.

I would also like to thank Isabel Clopp for her support, feedback and putting up with me; Vicki Paullin who has edited more of my work and made me believe I could be a writer; and Jason Shah who made the cover from drab to exciting. Jason used his talents to create a video that wound up on YouTube. Thanks to Carol Levin who has and is providing excellent marketing help plus editing. Thanks to Kandi Amelon for her fresh ideas and feedback.

This book was written with coffee bean stimulation provided by the wonderful baristas at Starbucks and Caribou. Thanks people and beans.

DISCLAIMER

This book is based solely on the opinions of Don Paullin for Fat Warriors, Inc. It is not based on scientific fact. It is not going to educate you on dieting, diet plans, or diet pills. We will not sell you pills or expensive plans. You can follow the Fat Warriors program for virtually no cost and it will pay off in huge, non-fattening dividends of smiley pride.

This book is not a guide on nutrition and does not take the place of medical help provided by physicians and other professionals. Don and Fat Warriors are neither nutritionists nor medical professionals. We do not give that type of advice and you should seek out these professionals as needed. Fat Warriors is based on the principles of behavior that will win for you.

Our presumption is that to follow this book you must have the basic judgment and education to know what is best for you. We are presenting a new and unique approach. Fat Warriors requires a paradigm shift of thinking that differs from easy, quick programs and miracle diets. Programs with before and after pictures seem to be right for those pictured, but never seem to work for anyone in achieving permanent change. If the pictures are your motivators, then stop reading and go take pictures. Fat Warriors is not for everyone, but it may be right for *you*. You decide.

Nothing in this book is based on scientific or dietary facts, plans, or pills. It seems that most diets, diet plans and pills fail, and are nothing other than clever marketing gimmicks. The Fat Warriors principles are based on common sense, and this book is completely different from others you will find on the topic.

So read, laugh, smile, cry, think, and then put on your War Face, growl, and fight fat!

TABLE OF CONTENTS

1

IT'S NOT OBESITY,
IT'S FAT UGLY

Public Enemy No. 1

The USA is at war with fat, and fat is winning by stacking American body counts. **Fat may be 10 pounds or 100 pounds, but in either case fat now controls much of America's waistlines.** In fact, nearly eight of ten adults become overweight at some point, and one-third of American adults are considered obese (30 pounds or more overweight). The current prevalence of fatness is so staggering, many consider it an epidemic. Fat is an ugly, mean killer that is devastating our nation's health, looks, and well-being. Nearly everybody knows somebody who has fallen to fat or is personally struggling and encased in fat's wrath.

Look around and you will see what politicians call obesity. "Obesity" is a kind, politically correct word. **I am at war and I call obesity *Fat Ugly* ("FU").** If you think FU means anything else, get over it. I am not kind to Fat Ugly because I hate how it looks on my family, my friends, and me. I hate that it surrounds you and makes you miserable.

Amnesty can be no option as fat is winning the war on thighs and hurting the eyes. The ultimate fat-fighting machine is the "Fat Warrior," Don Paullin. I intend to destroy FU, and I will not stop until the term Fat Ugly appears in the dictionary and obesity surrenders to Fat Warriors. Fat Warriors will win this fat war, so either join the Fat Warriors Nation and fight fat or sit on the couch and watch.

The Fat Warrior is determined to help fat adults and fat kids NOW. He wants to help you become your best personal Right Size of *Looking Good* ("LG"). This does not mean a model's body, but one that is right for <u>you</u>.

Don is not a nutritionist, doctor or dietician; he is a Warrior fighting fat. He does not believe diets work for the long term, and is on a mission to show you a better way to win your Best Bod and healthy lifestyle.

Which of the following statements is true when it comes to costing the government more in healthcare dollars?
- Obese people cost three times more than healthy people
- Obese people cost five times more than healthy people
- Obese people cost ten times more than healthy people
- Obese people cost the same as healthy people
- Healthy people cost the most

According to a report in *USA Today* (January 2008), research for the National Institute for Public Health and Environment found that healthy, thin non-smokers cost the most in healthcare dollars. Smokers and obese people died earlier, and therefore did not enjoy a longer life that racked up more healthcare costs! In healthcare dollars, healthy lifetime living costs $417,000; obesity costs $371,000; and smokers (who die prematurely) cost $326,000.

Is the message that you will die sooner and save the government money if you get fat and smoke?

YOU Are Not Fat Ugly!
It is important that you understand why *you* are not Fat Ugly. You are not Fat Ugly because your beautiful person inside is surrounded on the outside by layers of imprisoning fat. **Your Body Beautiful ("BB") is inside the layers and crying for help to get out.** The beautiful person resides inside to send pounding brain signals of painful depression, avoidance, health issues, and feeling horrible 24-7, hoping to be heard and freed. The beautiful person inside is screaming and wants out!

Hot Bods Everywhere
If you don't think fat is ugly, just look at a magazine. Magazines picture slender people, not fat people, because most people don't like to view pictures of fat people.

Pick up magazines, such as these, and you will see if fat people are pleasing to the eye: *People, Glamour, Vogue, In Style, Cosmopolitan, Vanity Fair, and Men's Health,* to name a few. Notice what body style is missing. Is it Fat Uglies or Hot Bods? Magazines are full of Hot Bods. **If the people shown in the magazines represented our actual population, you would think the United States lacked fat**

people. For the most part, there are no pictures of hoggers. The reason is simple: people do not pay to look at Fat Ugly. They prefer to see Looking Good people. That is reality, like it or not.

Look at the ads. They are loaded with beautiful people to get you to look at them. The big exceptions where you will find Fat Uglies are the ads for miracle diet plans, shakes, abs gadgets or other weight loss items that take you from before pictures to after pictures. They show the before Fat Ugly person, and then the same person looking totally hot after shaking off 80 pounds in 80 days with their shakes. What don't they show? Pictures of people after they pack on the rebound fat they've gained after stopping the programs or using the products.

Are you in a perpetual state of before, after, and then after the rebound?

Mad and Backed into a Corner

This book will tell you in brutally frank terms that there is nothing good or beautiful about being fat (possible exceptions being sumo wrestlers and polar bears). **This book is designed to embarrass you about your fatness, make you afraid of the fat life, and make you so mad that you want to go to war against your unhealthy fat and eliminate it.** We've written it to motivate you into becoming a member of the Fat Warriors Nation. You will join as a Recruit, advance to Private, Sergeant, and then progress to Fat Warrior status.

It is imperative that you start your fat war today and begin your fight. If you become a Fat Warrior, you will go to war to destroy your fat. You will have a War Face and a Combat Growl, and fat will fear you.

Become a Fat Warrior

The Fat Warrior is recruiting you to join his Army and stop the pandemic growth of obesity of all folks in our society. We are at war against fat in America, **with a vocabulary all our own.** We invite you to join us to defeat fat. We will give you the tools and teach you the methods you need to be successful. Together, let's start a revolution against fat!

Becoming a Fat Warrior is guaranteed to be challenging, but should lead you to a better, healthier lifestyle. In the end, you and your bod will feel and look victorious. You may achieve promotions and advance to Fat Warrior or even Drill Instructor status. You may then help your friends and family win their wars on fat. So, if you are ready for Fat Warriors boot camp, then be determined. Don't have onion skin. Do have alligator hide, put on your War Face, growl, and start marching through this book.

Steps to Become a Fat Warrior and Achieve Your Personal Right Size
- I am a Fataholic: Admit the Problem and Know the Pains
- Understand How and When Fat Ugly Imprisoned You
- What You Are Today Is Your Now: Know the Pain of Continuing Your Now
- Sell Yourself That Living a Fat Ugly Lifestyle Means War
- Turn Your Negative Emotions into Motivators for Victory
- Change Your Self-Talk and Beliefs Toward the New YOU
- Know Your Weapons of MassAssDestruction (WMAD)
- Lose Scale Detractors and Calorie-Counting Diverters to Achieve Your Personal Right Size
- ScoreBooking Is Quick and Easy: Record, Compare, Improve and Win Your Healthy Lifestyle
- Constantly Visualize Your Dreams
- Understand Why Turtle Speed Right Sizing Is Necessary
- Acknowledge Setbacks and Losses
- Celebrate Improvements and Joyous Victories
- Know Why Relapse Never Means Collapse
- Realize That Only Lifestyle Change Means Euphoric Victory
- Fight Fat One Decision at a Time, One Day at a Time, All the Time
- Give Up and Shut Up, or Fight
- Be Permanently Victorious

Fat Warriors Are NOT Politically Correct, nor Is Don
Politicians would take a politically correct approach to fatness, making it fine or at least okay to be fat. Some would then blame fat on corporate America, rich people, poor people, McDonald's, the media, the grocery store, and each other. Some would even tax fat. **Instead of the Flat Tax, we would have a Fat Tax.**

This book offers tough love, not PC-mistaken kindness for those who are plump sized. It provides fat-fighting techniques that work and discipline for making Body Beautiful decisions ("BBs"). It is also written with slender tongue in cheek.

Do you wonder why people eat too much? Political correctness makes it comfortable for people to be fat (or "horizontally challenged") and get fatter (or be a person of "substance"). Fat people must move out of their fat-cushioned comfort zones and fight to improve for health and happiness. You must hate your fatness, get mad, and fight to win your war against fat.

There are no marshmallows in this mess hall! If you want PC kindness, go to politicians. If you want sympathy, find your Mother. If you pretend fat is not hurting you, then take a trip to Disneyland. We will not treat Fat Ugly kindly or promise you that Right Sizing your bod will be easy or fast. It will be slow like the fable of the tortoise and the hare, but you will be the thinner winner in the long term with sustainable lifestyle results.

Last Warning, Onion Skins

If you have onion skin and a soft underbelly, then you may not want to find a solution to your fat problem, improve your health, and become fit. In that case, drop the book, grab the chips and dip into TV land. Only if you have alligator hide and can handle tough love should you proceed to joining the elite Fat Warriors Nation and go to war against Fat Ugly.

There is no feeling sorry for yourself. Fat Warriors means no entitlement mentality and NO WHINING. **WE DON'T TEACH WHINING, BLAME AND EXCUSES IN THIS BOOK.** We only allow whining and feeling sorry for yourself when talking to your priest, Mother or bartender.

Excuses work great for the person who believes them. We do not allow excuses to attend Fat Warriors boot camp. Can't Do is replaced with Can Do. Can-Do beliefs kick excuses' butts 100 percent of the time.

If you have a great excuse, keep it and lose this book. You do not want to proceed to Fat Warriors boot camp and teachings unless you are ready to fight. If you wish to make excuses and engage in Fat Ugly comfort behavior, then go to your Mommy and get some ice cream to feel better.

Notes

6

2

MOTIVATORS THAT KICK FAT'S ASS

Fat's Unconditional Surrender Is Your Looking Good Victory

Your Fat Warriors Drill Sergeant

I am your Fat Warriors Drill Instructor, D.I. Don. I fight ugly fat and want to help you become Body Beautiful ("BB"). I will be relentless in helping you fight Fat Ugly ("FU"). I am not nice! I will gouge fat's corpuscles, stomp on fat's cells, kick layers of fat ass, and cave the fat belly inward.

Fat Ugly is a murderer of people, money, sex, our nation's health and self-esteem. My mission is to eradicate fat and set people free. I am the ultimate fat-fighting machine and champion for a healthier, happier lifestyle. I am the Fat Super Hero without a cape and am the leader of the Fat Warriors Nation. Fat Warrior is what fat cells call me out of fear and respect. You may call me the Fat Warrior, and you may soon become a Fat Warrior.

Don Is Not:

The Fat Warrior is not skinny or even thin, but he is becoming his Body Beautiful slowly--one belt buckle hole at a time by following the steps outlined here. He is *that close* to his BB, and wants you to join him and be Body Beautiful too.

I will be relentless in helping you fight Fat Ugly (FU). I am not nice! I will gouge fat's corpuscles, stomp on fat's cells, kick layers of fat ass, and cave the fat belly inward.

This Is War!

The Fat Warriors mission is to fight fat, pledge to hate fat, and war excess fat off themselves, their families, and friends.

Fat Warriors do not promote skinny. We are at war for a healthy Right Size for ourselves and for those we love or care about. The goal is a new lifestyle that results in a happier, active life.

Whether you want to lose 10 pounds or 100 pounds permanently, the Fat Warriors principles will work for you.

Join the Fat Warriors Army As a Recruit

Like me, if you want to eradicate fat, you may join my Fat Warriors Army as a Recruit, advance to Private, then to Sergeant, until you achieve Fat Warrior status. You may also become a Fat Warrior D.I. That means you become a Drill Instructor and teach Recruits in boot camp to become Fat Warriors. To accomplish my dream, an Army in the *millions* will form the Fat Warriors Nation, winning Right Size freedom for the USA and beyond.

Advancement Ranks of the Fat Warriors

Volunteer: Anyone who helps a friend make better choices.

Recruit: Commits to learning the art of being a Fat Warrior.

Private: Trains to become a Fat Warrior. Has spent one month ScoreBooking and averaging FU and BB decisions and has shown improvement.

Sergeant: Completes three months of ScoreBooking and averaging. BB decisions outnumber FU decisions and show positive movement toward lifestyle changes. Total Can-Do attitude.

Fat Warrior: Pit-Bull determined mentality. Completes book one in the Fat Warriors series or attends a Fat Warriors boot camp seminar. Sustains a majority of BB decisions and demonstrates some lifestyle changes. Has taken the Fat Warriors oath and pledges to help others.

Drill Instructor: Helps and trains others to become Fat Warriors.

This Book Is Your Boot Camp

Think as though you are in Marine boot camp and the D.I. is preparing you for combat. During boot camp, you may cry, sweat, feel insulted, mistreated, feel stronger, experience pride, become a winner, and even laugh a lot. You will become prepared to be the ultimate FU-fighting machine. You may wish you were in band camp, but if you make it through boot camp you will be confident in your ability to destroy Fat Ugly. **If you make it through boot camp and graduate, you will be a Fat Warrior fighting fat and Looking Good, Feeling Good ("LGFG").**

Fat Warriors Boot Recruits Warning

Please understand that Fat Warriors boot camp is not for everyone, nor is the Fat Warriors philosophy. If at any time you feel you no longer want to participate, just put the book down and leave our camp. It is not a correct philosophy for everyone, just those whose needs it meets.

Don't feel bad if you can't make it as a Fat Warrior, but if you prevail you will unveil a happier lifestyle. **Your mind and body will change, and you will become a trained Fat Ugly fighter**. You will feel good, look good, and stand leaner. You will laugh, fare better with the opposite sex, feel stronger, be healthier, get high on life, and may even make more money.

It is well documented that many companies tend to favor people who are BB more than those who are FU. Talents being similar, which would you rather have representing you, a Fat Ugly or a Body Beautiful?

Fat Warriors Must Have a War Face, Combat Growl, and Fun!

Marines have a War Face and growl. Dogs and even puppies bare their teeth and growl, and it is scary. You must have a War Face and Combat Growl to scare fat and make it run off your hide.

Fat Warriors have a War Face, but they also have miles of smiles. They take themselves seriously, but never *too* seriously. **Our mission is serious for making people's lives better.** Put on your War Face, growl, and get started. Attention! Move out and read on.

Notes

10

3

I AM A FATAHOLIC

Admitting Fat Ugly Is Your Starting Line for Victory

Fat Warriors do not use scales to determine whether they are fat.

Are You Fat?

You only need to consult your mirror, your clothes, your belt buckle, and your mind for the answer. Your family or friends may diplomatically ignore your bulk bod or lie to you to avoid making you feel bad by embarrassing you. Friends that pretend not to notice are doing you a disservice. Whether it is 10 pounds or 100 pounds, you, your mirror and your belt will belt out the truthful answer to this question.

Who Determines if You Are Fat?

- That question should be answered, YOU DO. Fat Warriors demand honesty. Are you a dumpling? Determine if you are by taking this Fat Ugly Survey. (It's your survey, so whatever you say will be your truth.)
- Do you walk or *waddle*?
- When you stand on the scale, can you see your *toes*?
- Do your arms hang *outward* instead of straight down?
- Are you ordering your jeans like your meals-- *SuperSizeMyButt*?
- When people say you look *hot*, do they mean *overheated*?
- When the opposite sex refers to you as a *hunk*, do they mean *literally*?

11

- When the opposite sex says you have a *great ass*, do they mean *gigantic*?
- Would a masseuse give you a free massage or charge you *double*?
- Do you *cringe* when photographed?
- Do you require a *double seat* on a bus or airplane?

Send your humorous lines to www.FatWarriorsNation.com

The Fat Ugly Secret

Shush, whisper, be quiet. The Fat Ugly secret is that most fat people know they are imprisoned in layers of fat. You can't help yourself if you are not aware you are fat. You can only help yourself by recognizing your problem.

Fat people live with embarrassment and pain shared by family and friends who care. Society prefers to ignore it to spare feelings. Admitting it and talking about it is the way to find the solution, and the pain of being FU provides the motivation to win BB.

If you feel you are Fat Ugly and want to fight to change your life, you have taken the first step toward taking back your personal Right Size.

Are You Fat Ugly, Looking Good or Thin?

For the purpose of this book, there will be three body types only on the bod scale. It is true there are varying degrees of each body type, but we will not quibble appearances down into degrees. There is no scientific methodology behind this. It's as easy as one, two, and three to select your bod type. So be picky and pick out the body type you are and the one you want to be.

One key to your success is simply to be truthful. Answer the question to yourself. It must be an HONEST answer for you to improve. **You can never find the solution if you do not see the problem.** Fortunately, this problem is as big as you are and easy to spot. If you are not sure which body type you are, ask your family or friends to help you decide.

1. **Fat Ugly ("FU")**: FU means you are out at third; you will not score often. Look in the mirror and if you think and feel imprisoned in Fat Ugly, you probably are. FU is scoreless in all categories except misery.
2. **Body Beautiful ("BB")**: BB means never having to say you are fat or model thin. You will score more often in the happiness meter of life when you are BB. Body Beautiful scores the most. It is slightly above thin and is a very healthy-looking body as compared to skinny. Body Beautiful is eye candy with an active, healthy lifestyle.
3. **Thin**: Healthy thin also wins. Model thin may be in, but not with Fat Warriors. If you start looking like you just ran a marathon, unless you have, you may be going too far with thinness. Anorexia is a dangerous disease, so see a doctor for this problem, not the Fat Warrior. Thin is in, but only wins if it is a *healthy* thin.

   Fat is an ugly health disorder, too thin is an eating disorder. Both are unattractive and kill. They kill good looks, self-esteem, sex, the better jobs, and they can kill you.

Name & Claim Your Fat Uglies ("Fuglies")

- Grandma arm flappies
- Thigh-flapping clothes music
- Good butt has become fat ass
- Fat calves gone grazing
- Tummy isn't yummy
- Chins: more than one, less than 20
- Neck has turtled: no visible neck
- Fat Gut Strut is something you do
- Plus sizes fit fine

Add your favorite Fuglies with humor and send to www.FatWarriorsNation.com!

Notes

4

HOW YOUR BOD BECAME FAT UGLY

Blame Game: Top 10 Targets Blamed for Causing Fat Ugly

1. Fataurants
2. Foods to die for that kill--and they may, like sweet tooth treats such as hot fudge sundaes and candy bars.
3. Mother and/or Father
4. Chubby Genes from Mom, Dad & Gramps
5. Fat-Loving Friends
6. Television Couching and Chipping
7. Quitting Smoking
8. Job or Relationship Stress
9. Big Mac Attacks
10. Politicians

What do you blame most for your FU? Send to our website at www.FatWarriorsNation.com!

Blame Game

You can blame your fat on many things. Blaming allows you to feel good while feeling bad. The transfer of fat blame allows you to feel good by blaming while you are feeling bad about the reality of emotional drains caused by being Fat Ugly.

Defining the Problem
You do not have a weight problem
You do not have an eating problem
You do not have an exercise problem

You DO have a decision problem
You DO have a self-discipline problem
You DO have a lifestyle problem

Flash! Good News

The good news is that you do not have a weight problem. That's right! The extra weight you are carrying is perfect for the decisions you are making and the lifestyle you are living. **You do have a self-discipline and decision problem. Fix that and you fix you for life.**

James Bond Is You and You Are 008 with a License to Kill Fat

You are the doctor, you are the detective, and you are the keeper of the secret. Look back in time to your past, when you were BB or close to it. **To unlock your fat mystery, start thinking and be brutally honest with yourself**. What decisions did you make and follow at that time that made you FU? Did you grab grub on the go? Did you eat more than you thought? Did you sneak in snacks, samples and sweet treats? If you can visualize your decisions changing your Body Beautiful over to Fat Ugly, then you have started to solve your fat mystery. Write down your story in one or two pages. It is important to write this down for comparison in one year. **Don't doubt or pout. Just write your two pages now.**

You can be Sherlock Holmes <u>and</u> James Bond. You will solve the mystery and have a license to kill fat. Yes, James Bond is a Fat Warrior. Note how all the Bonds have BBs and get the girls. All the Bond females are also Fat Warriors--notice how they all have BBs and always get James Bond. You, too, can have your personal best BB and always get ...?

You have met, fingerprinted and finger pointed the FU enemy, and it is YOU!

Analyze WHO Made You FU

If you are fat, why are you fat? What caused you to get there? It is not "*what*," but rather "*who*." The answer lies with the fingerprints on your silverware and drinking glasses. **The knife in your back and the spoon digging your grave have YOUR fingerprints on them. The fork that is forking your path to diabetes and heart problems is YOURS.**

Fat Ugly is about YOU. That is great news, because it means YOU have the power to win your war on fat--so take control now!

GAME ON!
Don't feel sorry, get mad at Fat Ugly.
FU is personal, so let's go win your personal war on fat!

Notes

5

POUNDING OUT PROFITS BY THE POUND:

Diet Plans, Pills, Meals, Shakes, and Miracle Products

Lost and Found Rule:
I lost the fat, but fat found its way back in the same massive places.

Rebound Fat: The Revolving Problem

Are you tired of failing diets? Have you tried numerous diets and suffered rebound fat? **Whether you want to lose 10 pounds or 100 pounds permanently, the Fat Warriors principles will work for you.**

My Inspiration to Help You: A Friend's Story

My friend, who is overweight, told me that diet plans virtually destroy people with the yo-yo effect because they only work temporarily. He would lose 80 pounds on a program. His friends would compliment him and say he was Looking Good and standing tall. Then he would gain the Fat Ugly back, along with horrible depression plus the avoidance factor. He said, **"Tell people about the horrible depression that happens with rebound weight gain."**

My friend also told me about the avoidance problem. The avoidance problem happens when you gain back the weight you lost and become so depressed that you avoid going out or seeing your friends. This isolation adds to your angst and depression. I had no idea that my friend felt this way because he always seemed fat and jolly. He keeps up a positive attitude even though he is hurting under the fat façade. He is strong. My friend is also a former alcoholic who joined Alcoholics Anonymous (AA) and has not had a drink in 20 years. In addition, he quit smoking, proving he does have the **Willpower Howitzer** for fighting.

Anybody can lose weight. Most fat people have lost weight many times over the years. I estimate my friend has lost over 1,000 pounds in 25 years. He has proven he can lose weight and proven that he always gains it back.

If losing weight has little effect on the cause of your fatness, then you will likely gain it back. It is changing your lifestyle with bod-altering decisions that will help you sustain your personal Right Size permanently.

After the last diet plan, my friend resigned himself to be fat and said he would not try any more programs. All things combined had made him weak and he lost his will to fight. Diet plans just drained him emotionally and financially. That is when I decided to study Fat Ugly and find the answers. The genesis of Fat Warriors books and www.FatWarriorsNation.com began.

Easy Is for Selling Diets, Pills and Products

Becoming fat is pleasurable, and staying FU is easy greasy. Easy and fast is in all the ads for fad diets, diet pills, fat burners, shakes, and exercise machines. The easier they are the quicker you lose, **and** the faster the rebound weight returns. Toss in the best before and after pictures, free trial, and the sale is complete.

Ask fat waddlers how many diets, plans, pills, machines, and other products they have bought. Ask them! Count them! The question you must ask is why they failed. All the quick fixes are unnatural ways to take fat off and have one common problem--they do not work, or at best have the yo-yo diet effect.

Becoming a Fat Warrior is not associated with the word "easy." It is associated with a challenging, hard-earned lifestyle victory for a happier, healthier, sexier life. Only after winning your Looking Good, Feeling Good lifestyle will you find it compellingly easy!

Fat Warriors Riddle: If miracle plans are so easy and fast, why do the fat people last?

Fad Diets Make Money, Not Skinny

There should be a diet called *Lose Money, Not Weight--The Truthful Diet Plan. Just send us your money, sit on the couch, and let nothing happen. Good news, no rebound fat, you will just stay fat!*

Fad diets, diet books, diet pills, and diet meals are for separating people from their money, not from fat. You likely have heard the claims of these "revolutionary" products or items: lose 7 pounds in two days; lose 5-10 pounds per week for a month, then 3 pounds a week after that. There is the grapefruit diet, the carbohydrate cutter, the 20-meal plan program, metabolism boosters, and others. Maybe you have tried some of them. Did they work for you in the long term or even at all? Most likely, you are reading this book and joining Fat Warriors because everything else has failed you.

Realize that if any one of the fad diets contained the magic fat potion, there would be no fat people left. **Give them up or give up your money. It is the Fat Trilogy to be fat, broke, and stupid.** For any of you who are offended by the term "stupid," the Fat Warrior apologizes. Please, just because you lost your money instead of your pounds, you don't have to lose your sense of humor. Take off your pounds and put on your sense of humor.

Delete Key Dieting

When you are on a diet program, taking diet pills, or consuming some other quick-loss product, it may seem as easy as hitting the delete key to make Fat Ugly disappear. However, unlike computer files, you can't simply delete your fat. Unfortunately, the fat is only going to your body's recycle bin and will show up again later on when you have stopped using the product. Some of these products and programs may be dangerous as well, and there is often no real evidence to support their claims other than before and after pictures. How many of those do you need to see?

You cannot delegate the responsibility of your body to any program or product, no matter what they claim. **You own your bod for good or bad.** You have the accountability for it. **What**

happens to your bod happens on your watch. Don't try to shift and lose the responsibility for your bod to diets, pills or meals on wheels, shakes, fat bombers, or fat blasters. Fad diet and weight loss products companies provide false hopes and fat profits. They are more interested in their bottom line than your bottom. Are you bottomed out on them?

Diet programs get you to depend on them as they depend on your wallet.

Meals on Wheels

Got your meals coming on wheels to your house? You can eat lasagna, cheeseburgers, pizza, and wow, order now! Bringing you easy prepared meals on wheels probably works if you only eat THEIR food and THEIR microscopic portions for life. The question you must ask is whether that is a lifestyle change that you will be comfortable with forever. If it is not sustainable, then when the wheels come off the pounds return.

Meals on wheels plans and other special meal programs claiming to help you lose weight also come with sticker shock. The expense for a one-month supply usually costs hundreds of dollars.

Changing your fat tire is not as easy as changing an auto tire. However, it is much easier than riding on the rim. Continuing to ride on a fat tire, like riding on the rim, will destroy your performance. Jack it, change it, and move on!

Buns of Steel

Did anybody ever get buns of steel? I think Superman and Wonder Woman might have buns of steel. It must be hard to sit with buns of steel. Do buns of steel shine or clank? Ask Clark.

Six-Pack Abs

I have six-pack abs, but they are from drinking six packs for many years. I think my idea of six-pack abs has a largely different shape on my stomach, and my buns of steel are rusting.

Fat Warriors No-Cost Plan

Usually high quality comes at high cost, low quality at low cost. Most diet pills and products are low quality but high cost. Fat Warriors is luxurious quality at low cost!

You can win your Body Beautiful for nothing down and nothing in the future. There is no fee to start making BB decisions, but you must make an investment in yourself. There are no meals, no wheels, no pills, and no calorie points. We have no guarantee since fat warring can have no cost. Your first week can be free, as can all the other weeks and years. Yes, get your first year free, and the next 99 years too!

It is easy to guarantee your money back for a no-cost plan. We do offer products, books, seminars, and are developing more methods to provide training, inspiration, education, and fun to the Fat Warriors Nation. You can do all this on your own, but we add the fun, inspiration, and educational tools at minimal cost. For more information and updates, please visit our website at www.FatWarriorsNation.com!

Notes

6

TURNING FAT EMOTIONS INTO LEAN DREAM MOTIVATORS

Emotional Pains Can Help Defeat Your Fat Ugly

Salesmanship, the First Step from FU to BB

The most important initial step in fat loss is salesmanship. **The reason you are Fat Ugly is that you are a poor salesperson. As long as you can't sell yourself on fighting for your personal Right Size, you will remain FU. You must sell yourself on paying the price for your Body Beautiful.**

You thought the first thing would be something about counting calories, fat grams or scale weighing. Nope. Put first things first. You must first sell yourself on the fact that you are fat. Not only are you fat, but also *Fat Ugly*. Ouch, Fat Ugly hurts! Do you dislike how you look in that tight-fitting clothing? Do you feel bad about your appearance? Do you wish you could improve your body image, health, and self-esteem? Is Fat Ugly appropriate?

That FU hurt provides motivation to fight. You must have and need that pain to strongly feel the determination to make decisions that will evolve into healthy lifestyle changes.

You must sell yourself on the secret salespeople know, which is that **PEOPLE BUY THINGS BASED ON EMOTIONS, NOT LOGICAL FACTS.** This understanding will allow you to transform the painful emotions like embarrassment and depression into motivational muscle. **The more Fat Ugly hurts and makes you go from depression, to anger, then MAD, the better the odds that you will pay the price to win BB. MAD wills fighting back!**

Cognitive Dissonance: The Difference Between What You Have and What You *Want*!

Cognitive dissonance is the difference between what you have and what you want. Mirror yourself right now for your cognitive dissonance. *While you look like this now, do you want to look like this for 10, 20, or 30 years? When you think about this, it is a horrifying life sentence.* People act for change only when they reach a pain threshold of cognitive dissonance. If you experience the pain of cognitive dissonance, you can start making winning decisions right now and win one decision at a time for your lifetime of more smiles, happiness, and health.

Magic Moment

Wow, this Fat Ugly cognitive dissonance is sad and an emotionally depressing evaluation when you are fat. On the other hand, you can see clearly what you want and turn it into your magic moment. **Your magic moment is when you decide that you want to become your personal Right Size so bad that you will fight and make the BB decisions necessary to attain it.** Know your cognitive dissonance, feel the pain, and pain will motivate you to change to win the lifestyle you deserve.

Cognitive dissonance is the difference between what you have and what you want. **Ask yourself, "What is my cognitive dissonance?"**

Cognitive Dissonance Examples:

- Fat Ugly unattractiveness vs. Body Beautiful attractiveness
- The bod you see vs. the bod you want, plus the joys and health it will bring
- Emotional embarrassment with your FU bod vs. the proud euphoric joy you can achieve with your BB
- The unhealthy dangers of Fat Ugly vs. the healthy lifestyle benefits of Body Beautiful
- Pills vs. treadmill
- Dating down Fat Ugly vs. dating up Body Beautiful
- Avoiding vs. participating
- Fat clothes vs. cool clothes
- Fat Ugly lifestyle vs. Looking Good, Feeling Good lifestyle

---

Think of your cognitive dissonance examples
and list your Top 10. Share them on
www.FatWarriorsNation.com!

Emotional Pain: Your Best Motivator

Feel your pains. Feel the pain of being Fat Ugly. Feel the pain of not getting the best selection of the opposite sex because you are a blimp. Feel the pain of not getting that job even though you know you are the most qualified, but lost because you were seen as a pig. The pain of how you physically feel from carrying all that fat around every day. The pain of trying to avoid people because of your whale belly and hippo hips. Fear that you may be heading toward health problems like diabetes, cancer, and heart disease. **The shame and embarrassment of being FU will provide extra self-motivation to get you to learn how to use the Fat Warriors weapons.**

Is the pain unbearable? If it is, that is great because you can turn emotional pain into self-motivation. If not, keep heaping on the pain, as it will motivate and help set you in motion to become BB. Are eating the goodies so great that you are willing to endure these emotional pains?

Think about your pain and compare that with feelings of Looking Good, Feeling Good 24-7. Looking Good and Feeling Good with the wonderful seasoning taste of high self-esteem and positive energy. LGFG means having people compliment you instead of gawking at your Fat Ugly frame. LGFG means being able to fit into the clothes you love.

Is the malt, the SuperSizeMyButt meal, the pig-out eating, the inactivity, and the late-night snacking worth the pain of wearing them forever? **Do you want others to know you as Fat Ugly, or are you ready to win your Right Size war instead?**

If you feel like crying, feel sad, feel sorry, and feel depressed, that is great. That emotional pain is your "must" motivation to make your decisions for change. Your FU pain will now become an extra self-motivator muscle to help you win your war.

Feel the pain; I mean *really* feel the pain and make it work for you.

Fear

Fear can paralyze you into no action or it can cause positive fighting action. It can save your life. Fear of Fat Ugly can be the best motivator to win that there is.

Fear. Understand it, live it, and let it compel you to fight like a pit bull--relentless and unyielding to fat pleasures. The fear of being Fat Ugly for life may stop you from eating ice cream or a SuperSizeMyButt meal. Fear may cause you to take action and be your own ally. This is Fat Ugly fear. You must possess FU fear to win your war against fat.

What do you fear? Do you fear your peers talking behind your back about your fatness? Do you fear people staring at you as you pile extreme amounts of food onto your plate at the buffet? Do you fear a triple bypass because of your clogged arteries or not fitting into your clothes?

Most of my success in endeavors goes with the dream of the benefits of success. However, sometimes the fear of losing a promotion or a job motivated me to go that extra mile. Fear of going broke in business caused me to work extra hard and long hours to enjoy success. Fear of failure in public speaking motivates me to prepare so that I do not die on stage. The hard-core results: Controlled fear may be good if it works for your success.

Fear may cause you to make BB decisions that save your arteries and your life. You can wallow in the fear of never Looking Good and Feeling Good, or fight for your LGFG lifestyle. Let your fears be a war weapon for you.

Embarrassment is akin to fear and will either help you win your Body Beautiful, or help you find excuses to feel sorry for your fat self.

Neither pity nor sympathy will help you win. They will only help you feel good feeling bad. Feeling good feeling bad is not good.

Embarrassment

If you own Fat Ugly, you think constantly of what people think of you when you walk into a coffee shop, restaurant, school, the movies, or anywhere. You wonder if they are looking at you and what are they thinking as they watch you hogging down that barrel of buttery FatCorn, large soda, candy, and more at the movie theater. Do you look more forward to greasy FatCorn than the movie?

People see you and wonder if you can squeeze into a seat with comfort, and where do you buy those huge jeans? They look at your FU body as you swallow the FatCorn and hose it down with a gigantic sugar drink. As you sit and shovel the warm, buttery kernels into your fat face, how do you feel? **If you feel embarrassment, then you can use it as motivator muscle to win BB.** If you don't feel the embarrassment, then you have probably given up defeated. Put the book down and pick up the chip dip.

Fat Warriors Law:
The chances of winning your personal war on fat are directly proportional to your pain levels of owning Fat Ugly. The higher your pains of being fat, the higher your chances of defeating FU permanently. Understanding the embarrassment you feel, the scariness of facing health issues, and the thought of not being a good dating or mating prospect will help you fight back. The more these things hurt, the more they motivate you to fight and defeat. So put on your War Face, growl, and fight your Fuglies!

In addition to being overweight, I was once a smoker. Uncool. Standing outside of a smoke-free building while people walked by raised my self-stupid and embarrassment level. This constantly reminded me of how stupid I was for smoking, and I constantly tried to quit. Smoking made me look ugly and I was embarrassed. I called it Smoking Ugly to myself. Smoking was socially unacceptable, expensive, and gave me bad breath. There is not much on the positive side of smoking. It made me feel totally embarrassed about smoking and about not having the self-discipline to make the decision to quit and execute it.

After hearing enough criticism, negative talk and feeling embarrassed, I finally decided I would never smoke again. It was one of my longest, hardest battles, but I did it. Embarrassment was a key pain motivator muscle, and Pit-Bull mentality to stop was the winning blow.

Hurt

Finding love can be hard for those who carry around all that extra fat. The dating pool for Fat Ugly people is reduced because their size is not. FUs are just not the date of choice for most BBs. Fair or not, it shows how bad it is for Fat Ugly people and the hurt and pain they must endure. **Hurt can be a powerful motivator muscle to win your fat war.**

Law of Dating Pool:
Your dating pool is reduced in direct proportion to the amount of fat you've produced.

7

WEAPONS OF MASSASSDESTRUCTION (WMAD)

Fat Ugly Is the Enemy

Fat Warriors Pledge

Only I can win MY war against MY fat. My BB decisions are my weapons against FU. My decisions will set free my Body Beautiful currently imprisoned by Fat Ugly.

My decisions will be with me when pills, fad diets, and wheel meals are gone. I will keep making BB decisions until they become a lifestyle change. I will become a Fat Warrior, and I will recruit my friends and family to join the Fat Warriors Nation.

True or False?

Candy bars, hot dogs, ice cream, pastries, large portions, and Fataurants make me fat.

Answer: False. It's *decisions* that make you fat.

Disciplined Decisions Are Fat Bullets

Fat Warriors understand that they eat decisions that look like food, but are actually critical decisions put into and onto the bod. It is important that you look at food as *decisions*.

Decisions are your secret weapons that will kick fat's ass. FU decisions have been making you fat. Really, it's just decisions that are making me fat, not food? Yep. You thought it was the candy bars, doughnuts, ice cream, or MochaChocaLattes. Nope, it was the decisions that put them within reach and then into your mouth.

Fatal Distractions

Great News! Your ability to make Body Beautiful decisions is with you every waking moment of the day and totally under your control. Changing from FU decisions to BB decisions starts out hard, and then gets easier as they become habit or lifestyle, along with willpower. **There are no fatal distractions of excuses, blame game, counting calories, or looking at scales. It is all about decisions and choices, two magic bullets in the arsenal of Fat Warriors.**

Your Missile Can't Miss

Before you are armed with the Fat Warriors equivalent of a nuclear block-busting, fat-killing missile, you must be armed with intel (intelligence). Intelligence shows that human behavior is naturally goal oriented. That means you will constantly try to improve if you measure and seek an obtainable goal. Your very own self-motivated missile can't miss.

The guidance system of your can't-miss missile is your thoughts. Your thoughts will signal the knife, the fork, and the drinking glass as to the choices they can move into your mouth.

Your Brain: The Fat Warriors Ultimate Fighting Weapon

You are in Fat Warriors boot camp and are entitled to your own command center. Your personal command center goes by the code name **BRAIN**. Your brain is ready and willing to provide you with support and strategic fat war planning upon immediate notice 24-7. You program it and tell it what you want to do and it will help you. It will supply any weapon needed to help you win your war against Fat Ugly, such as providing you with the confidence and courage to help you stare down an ice cream cone.

The brain controls your eyes, tongue, mouth, stomach, and heart. You trigger your command center with every decision you make. Your brain is either your Fat Warriors ultimate weapon or the cannon turned against you.

Your personal command center is wireless, tireless, invisible, and invincible. No one else can see your stealth command center or hear it because it is uniquely yours. You can only win if you use your brain to make the right decisions and never give up. The brain plan is free, untaxed, with unlimited minutes. Like MasterCard, it is priceless.

The brain will naturally start making more BB decisions and fewer FU decisions if you give it a goal target. This creates positive momentum and reinforcement of your good decisions.

You Must Be at War with Fat, Not McDonald's, to Win

Do you want to destroy Fuglies and keep them off you and your family? **If so, see your FU decisions as the enemy, not fat foods.** It is not McDonald's burgers, fried or fast foods, desserts or pizza that made you own Fat Ugly. It's the DECISIONS you made to eat Fugly foods rather than their healthier counterparts, like grilled or baked choices, fruit, vegetables, whole grains, and other good foods. Fugly foods are innocent until you put them on your taste buds, swallow and allow them in your bod and mind. Yes, they are in your mind also!

The Business Meeting Food-A-Thon

If you are a business person seeking that LGFG look, then you will definitely want to put up your best defense at your next business function. Eat Free is often the appeal at many business gatherings. At these events, business people often stand around a big buffet table filling their plates repeatedly with greasy appetizers, pastries, high-fat deli meat, fried side dishes, plus beverages--none of which they have to pay for, which makes it all the more tempting to keep treating and eating.

Fat Warriors know the real cost of free food at meetings. It surely will not lead to leaner limbs and a flatter tummy. Instead, join your smarter-thinking business pals at the veggie tray (skip the creamy dip) and get some bottled water. The fun is not in the indulging, but in living the fun life.

Use Your Weapons of MassAssDestruction

We are at war. You are in boot camp to become a Fat Warrior and are ready for training to utilize the weapons of MassAssDestruction.

You will align all of your weapons for one great fat-killing machine: **your brain, decisions, self-motivation, discipline, emotions, beliefs, accountability, and lifestyle changes.** These are the keys that drive this program.

Pit-Bull Mentality:
You are at war with your FU decisions. Your mission as a Fat Warrior is to seek and destroy Fuglies and take no prisoners.

8

FantaSizing while eating naked

FantaSizing Eating Naked

There are three levels of Eating Naked and they all deal with stripping bare. The first is stripping yourself of all your old eating habits, thoughts, and ideas about how and what you should do to be in control of your eating behaviors. The second is beginning to strip away the chemicals and additives in the food you eat by learning to shop and eat organic. The third may be the most fun, depending on who you do it with and the fantasies you have when you do it. **This is actually Eating Naked.**

The first step in Eating Naked starts with the decision to eat more chemical-free and fertilizer-free foods, limiting processed foods such as white bread, and selecting more organic foods. Adding chemicals possibly adds more Fuglies and fat addictions than calories.

Eating Naked and FantaSizing while doing it can be pleasurable and fun with positive rewards. Eating Naked while FantaSizing may carry a Mature Rating and should only be done by consenting adults. It can be done in the kitchen, dining room, and even the bedroom. The foreplay starts in your mind and is executed at the grocery store or market!

I always FantaSize while Eating Naked. My fantasies are made up of positive visions of how and what I want my bod and lifestyle to be. It is fun and easy. I Eat Naked and FantaSize about a firmer bod and sexy flat stomach.

Eating Naked is easy to get used to and grows on you as you accomplish the goals of an energetic lifestyle of slimness. It is thinking about Looking Good, Feeling Good ("LGFG").

Atom Bombs of FatCrap

FatCrap is defined as undesired additives and chemicals placed into processed foods. **FatCrap is an ugly name for ugly chemicals.**

There may be an atom bomb inside of you that is blowing you up to fatness. Atoms of microscopic chemicals may be mutating you into Fat Ugly.

Chemicals may cause fruits and vegetables to plump up quickly and make cattle, poultry, and pigs fatter faster for slaughter. Might you be becoming plumper or fatter faster because of these same chemicals? These chemicals are used to grow, plump up, fat up, preserve, and do things to foods that are not natural. They may be called things like hormones, steroids, preservatives, and fertilizer. I just call ugly chemicals FatCrap that may be SuperSizing you. These FatCrap chemicals may be labeled with names you cannot pronounce or define.

You may be putting FatCrap undesirables into your body without even knowing their harm. These are chemicals you are putting into your body that nature neither intends nor desires for your healthy bod and mind.

Stripping Naked Eating

Stripping Naked means undressing your foods and removing toxic chemicals from your bod. Organically stripping your foods of all FatCrap chemicals is great for body, mind, and spirit. Eating Naked is called "eating clean" or "organic" by some, and this means eating pure food without added chemicals.

I call washing my food "eating clean," and so I prefer the term Eating Naked. Whatever you call it, many experts agree that by Eating Naked or clean you will expose your bod to healthier foods, and as a result become smaller and healthier. Your mind will also be stripped clean of those negative toxins that may cause depression and suppress your best health.

Nudist Naked

There are two types of people who Eat Naked. Nudists are the first group of Naked Eaters. Nudists strip themselves of chemicals found in foods by reading labels, disrobing FatCrap-laden foods, and removing them from their palates. You can spot a nudist at the grocery store reading labels, putting FatCrap foods back on the shelf, and buying only foods that are stripped clean.

The second type of Naked Eater is the organic purist. Organic purists don't read labels. Instead, they select foods from the certified organic section only. They eat certified organic food and here is how ingredients are listed on these labels:

- Almond package: Ingredients Almonds
- Carrot package: Ingredients Carrots
- Steak package: Ingredients Beef

This explains why organic purists do not need glasses to read labels, as the text does not have to be small.

Have you ever thought about how to practice the art of Eating Naked?

Expose Your Body

Exposing yourself to real food as nourishment without FatCrap may be more powerful than counting calories. If you Eat Naked, many other positive things will happen for you, and counting calories and standing on scales may become ghosts of the past.

Chemical Free for Me?

We are not suggesting that you must go entirely chemical free! **Fat Warriors believe that you should look at organic and fresh eating as part of your lifestyle.** You must decide how chemical free you want to be. Fat Warriors want you to consider what is right for you and recommend experimenting by reading labels and buying some organic foods as a starting point.

If chemicals are making plants plumper and pigs fatter faster, are these chemicals doing the same to you? Preservatives keep foods preserved for longer periods than nature provides. Nature spoils natural foods more quickly to prevent us from eating bad food.

Eating fresh foods that are grown locally and products from grass-fed animals will eliminate many bad chemicals. Going chemical free may help you obtain your best nourishment, your best mood, best health, and provide you with your personal best Body Beautiful to show off.

Dip your toes in the water, try a few things, and see if the idea grows on you!

Notes

9

SLOW DOWN! TURTLE SPEED WINS YOUR RIGHT SIZE FOREVER

Are you in it for life? Then slow and steady will beat the quick fad diets every time for your lifetime.

Law of Slow Is Faster:
The amount of time it takes for you to take weight off quickly may be approximately the amount of time it will take you to gain it back. The slower it comes off, the longer it stays off. You are not in a hurry to Right Size. Your only focus is making decisions for permanent lifestyle changes.

Fat Warriors Speed Is Slow, Then Slower!

We want you to **lose weight slowly, and then even slower, and eventually be able to stop as you near your personal Right Size**. You will understand the story *behind* the rabbit and our Fat Warriors turtle. The rabbit wanted easy, quick weight loss, and took off at full speed to win the race. He tired quickly with easy plans and easy pills. He ran out of breath and could not find Will Power. The rabbit quickly lost weight and then experienced rebound fatness by the pounds, unable to make it to the finish line.

The turtle preferred making permanent lifestyle changes, and planned a sustainable victory instead of a race. The turtle remained constant and true to his beliefs and never rebounded with pork-up pounds. The rabbit under-ate and then over-ate, got fat, and could not run the entire race. The rabbit lives in Waddle Beach, Florida today and works as a whale. That is the way the Fat Warriors tell the rabbit and turtle story with glory. Warrior is our turtle's name, and Warrior is the winner!

For any program or exercise to work, it must be sustainable. Sustainability is the key to lifestyle changes, and lifestyle changes are the key to driving around in your best Hot Bod forever.

Self-Reliant Sustainability

Our turtle's mantra is self-reliant *sustainability.* **The behavioral changes you make, whether portions, selection of food or exercise, must be sustainable to be maintainable.** Non-sustainable is rabbit speed, but the rabbit can't run full speed for the long run. Self-reliant sustainable behaviors that become lifestyle changes develop over time and can be permanent.

In a television show, contestants rapidly drop large numbers of pounds per week. They seem to work out in the gym all day, have a personal trainer, eat only controlled foods, and don't go to work. How is that **sustainable?** Unsustainable lifestyle changes likely mean rebound weight gain. **Sustainable lifestyle changes more likely give you permanent results.**

Why Turtle Speed Beats Rapid Rabbit Weight Loss

It may not be biologically correct, but in southern Kansas where I grew up, we called a tortoise a turtle. I also never saw a cowboy go hare hunting. We all learned to hunt rabbits. Hare stew would just not sound as good as rabbit stew.

Since I am the Fat Warrior, I will tell you why we believe turtle speed Right Sizing will beat the rabbit's speedy weight loss approach every time. **A slower pace may be directly proportional to the success of permanent lifestyle changes.**

The more slowly fat comes off, the longer it stays off. If lost quickly, then it usually returns quickly.

The faster the weight loss, the fatter it comes back. All the motivational ads show people before and after in a short time span. There are pictures of Fat Ugly people before, and then after miraculously transforming into a Hot Bod in 60 days. Go on their plans, shakes, pills, special meals, and you will lose. Guaranteed. The rabbit weight loss is quick and it works as long as you follow their programs.

The clue to failure is the quickness of taking pounds off, because it is probably not sustainable. Let's say you lose the weight rabbit quick by relying on a miracle program. Once that ends, then the onus is right back where it should be--on YOU. If it is not sustainable behavior, you return to your old habits and gain the weight back. That is because it is not your programmed lifestyle.

You put on and wear your yo-yo weight gain once again, minus your skinnier wallet. However, it is your fault and the proof is on your butt.

Think Slow

Think about gaining a winning lifestyle for the long term. Fat Warriors don't diet, don't starve, don't do shakes, don't carb or not carb, and don't deprive.

Fat Warriors simply keep increasing BB decisions and decreasing FU decisions as a part of their lifestyles over time. We eat everything in moderation, like red meat, chicken, fish, good fats, carbohydrates, veggies, and even occasionally junky chunkies and fat snacks. **Fat Warriors are not movie stars, but aspire to our best personal Hot Bods, not skinny bods. However, it takes time.**

Tip: Increase BB decisions and decrease FU decisions as a part of your lifestyle over time. Eat everything in moderation, like red meat, chicken, fish, good fats, carbohydrates, veggies, and even occasionally junky chunkies and fat snacks.

Envision Your Right Size, Not Weight Loss

Say no to losing weight and say yes to Right Sizing. Making fewer Fuglies will result not in downsizing, but in *Right Sizing* your bod. There is no wonderful vision in losing weight, only dread, but there are abundant pleasures with Right Sizing.

Envision Right Sizing and driving around in your Hot Bod. We are talking handsome, beautiful figures, money figures, health, wealth, and esteem. Many wonderful visions come with Right Sizing. So focus on Right Sizing, not downsizing. **We are after the right weight, not weight loss. However, more importantly, a sustainable weight by making lifestyle changes over time.**

Here are a couple of examples from my own experiences: I failed quitting smoking for 25 years but I never gave up trying. I just kept quitting until the 26th year, and then I made it. Now my lifestyle is pain free, never thinking about smoking.

I was an ice creamaholic. I craved it and would order the largest malt available and drink it quickly until gone. My girlfriend, Cutie, would order a smaller malt, only drink half of it and put it in the fridge to finish later. Cutie's half-malt would awaken me in my sleep and call me to it. I would go down to the fridge and down the remaining malt. I not only had to wear the half-malt, but explain to Cutie that some pathetic, no-willpower-malt-stealer had robbed her.

It took time, but with Cutie's help I am ice cream free and have it about six times per year. We do not trust me and never keep ice cream in the fridge, the house, or in the neighbors' houses. I now have a lifestyle of little ice cream, but more importantly I do not miss it.

Tip: Start making a behavior change and in about 30 days it becomes a lifestyle. The pain of change goes away as you develop your new lifestyle. You will be styling pain free in your Body Beautiful.

Are You a Swinger?

My coach in baseball taught us to shorten our swings when we had two strikes. A shortened swing allowed more control and made it more likely to get a hit, or put the ball in play and not strike out. The home run was a bad bet after two strikes.

When we are Fat Ugly, sometimes we feel like we have two strikes against us and we are thinking strikeout again. It may be best to shorten your swing and not try for losing 80 pounds in 80 days. Instead, take your time and just try to get a base hit. The shortened swing is a great bet for success and is more doable than hitting a home run.

Just start out with a base hit as one good decision replacing a bad one. Your base hits will become grand slam homers of sustainable lifestyle changes over time.

Notes

10

SCORING DETERMINES BBs AND FUs

Scoring Motivates Winners

Discover Your Triple Crown Jewels of Life

Just as in other areas of life, keeping track of your decisions score on a daily basis will naturally provide you with self-motivation to Right Size. Recording decisions is easy fun. We will show you the way to discover a scoring treasure chest filled with the jewels of your new envisioned lifestyle. You will be on your way to:

- looking your best
- feeling your best
- creating euphoric feelings
- tracking and seeing the results in your ScoreBook and in the mirror
- having your best health
- attaining optimum income
- enjoying your best life possible

It is a key concept that without keeping sports scores, few would play, fewer would watch, and nobody would win! You will see why ScoreBooking provides the self-motivation to win your war on Fat Ugly.

Become Your Personal Right Size by Keeping Score

Have you ever bowled a 300 game, a 200 game, or how about your first 100 game? Have you ever broken par or broken 100 in golf? Have you ever played baseball, tennis, or any game? Have you ever owned a business? **These activities involve keeping score, which optimizes the self-motivation and discipline to improve or win.** Without scoring, there would be no winners, losers, tournaments, games, or championships. Without records and scorekeeping, few athletes would be motivated to improve. Without scoring, there would be no records and we know that records are made to be broken--just like your rebound fat cycle.

In the game of golf, you want a low score to win. In bowling, you want a high score and consequent high average. When you record that great game, it is on the card for show and tell for the world to see. Businesses keep score on an income statement. When you record your first profits, big smiles are generated as people look at and share the positive scored results. Keeping score in business is so important it has its own name, and we call it the *bottom line*. **The point is that winning usually involves the keeping of scores to demonstrate success or progress.**

People even score in the dating game. Baseball players run around the bases and record a score. Scoring can signal success and is necessary for motivation, fun, and improvement. ScoreBooking puts the excitement and fun in the game, and leads to your Right Size.

ScoreBooking: The Must Way to Your Right Size

Do you want to lose wide hide permanently? Keep score! Need the self-motivation for making decisions to exercise and eat right? Then keep your score! Need the self-discipline to make decisions not to eat candy bars or other Fuglies? Then ScoreBook it!

The concept is that scoring is a natural self-motivator for competitive improvement. This means that if you do it, you will automatically improve YOU. Unlike programs you have tried in the past where the plans provide the motivation and the plans are in control, as a Fat Warrior you will be self-motivated and in total control.

Weight loss that is not permanent becomes rebound fat. The fact is that losing weight can be easy, but sustaining it is not. Achieving and maintaining your personal Right Size requires self-motivation and self-discipline. **Making great decisions and ScoreBooking them means less jiggle in your wiggle.**

Pain Week is a week to realize that what you have become affects your core of body, mind, and spirit.

Pain Week and Fabits

Your first week as a Fat Warriors recruit is Pain Week. This week is your starting line of ScoreBooking and reflecting on your weaknesses and Fat habits ("Fabits"). It is your week of recognizing why and how your bod grew to FU. It is not a week of guilt, but a week of understanding. It is a week to experience the pains of owning Fat Ugly. It is time to determine how FU affects your feelings, mood, social life, participation, career, health, wealth, and self-esteem.

A Week to Peek

Pain Week is seven days of opening your eyes to see the effects of your Fat Ugly lifestyle. What you normally eat and drink likely is what began your FU journey a long time ago. During Pain Week, note in your ScoreBook what you eat and the amount you consume. Also, note the amount of exercise, or lack of it.

Pain week is about feeling the pain, identifying and understanding what causes your current decisions that keep you imprisoned in Fat Ugly. When it is over, you have completed the first step to becoming a Private in the Fat Warriors Army.

P.S. Those who skip Pain Week and just start into recording based on memory of their history (routine) may do so without being sent to the Brig.

Feeling FU Pain Is Your Catalyst to Change

You will not change unless the pain is sufficient to cause you to pay the price to get what you want. **Buying your Body Beautiful and the health-esteem and self-esteem that goes with it requires paying the price of changing decisions and lifestyle.**

Just as in jobs and sports, with Fat Warriors decisions are made and performance scored. ScoreBooking is the only way you can tell if you are improving, winning, or losing. Keeping a record of your decisions provides absolute recognition of the good and the bad, and is the catalyst for the self-motivation and discipline needed to win the Right-Sized bod you can now only dream about.

Benchmark Musts for Gaining Your Personal Right Size

Benchmarks are a must for Right Sizing. To create benchmarks you must record scores of improvement. Grades cause people to study, gold medals cause people to train, money causes people to work harder, and bonuses cause people to out-perform goals. In each case, scores are kept, recorded, compared, and supply needed self-motivation.

If you are determined to win your war, you must score and compare your decision benchmarks. Do that and you will start making more positive decisions, which will turn your dream size into reality. Recording and comparing scores is mandatory to show your progress and optimize your success. **Do you want your new lifestyle? Then you must keep score. ScoreBooking works!**

Lie to Yourself and You Will Lie in Fat Ugly

The truth will set you free, but it will also help you win your war against Fat Ugly. Scoring must be done truthfully. If you lie about your decisions, the only person you will cheat and deceive is yourself. Your lies will keep you lying in fat forever. It is human to make mistakes, but be honest and record the truth. Honesty will keep you improving.

Never Quit Scoring and You Never Lose

You may become discouraged and think you can't do it. Never quit, but recommit to resume ScoreBooking. **You cannot lose if you are determined to fight and score.** It may take many attempts and time, but it is a necessary process for improving what is necessary for victory. Experiencing some failures is normal, but you will get back up and keep striving so you won't be defeated again!

11

YOUR SCOREBOOK MADE QUICK AND EASY

The Fat Warriors ScoreBook may alone cause more permanent success than all fad diets, miracle pills or other programs combined.

ScoreBooking: The Powerful Secret to Your Permanent Right Size

- Carry your Fat Warriors **ScoreBook** with you at all times for convenient anytime recordings. I suggest scoring once daily.
- Use your **ScoreBook** to plan, record and optimize your FU and BB decisions. See the improvements in averages.
- Once a day record your FU and BB decisions in your **Scorebook**. It is easy and quick, and you can do this in less than one minute. That's right, it takes less than 60 seconds a day to **ScoreBook** your decisions!
- Did you miss a day or two of recording your decisions? No problem! Just start **ScoreBooking** again. Missing is not important as long as you start recording and averaging again.
- We will explain how to calculate your BB Average and Fatting Average in your **Scorebook** to optimize your natural competitive spirit to make more BB decisions. You can do this in two minutes or less.
- Your Fat Warriors **ScoreBook** will help you achieve your goals for the Looking Good, Feeling Good Promised Land. **ScoreBooking** will leave you feeling proud and healthy when you have attained the level of behavior that is sustainable for you.

- **ScoreBooking** is not an option, but a must for optimum results. Scorebooking provides encouraging self-motivation and discipline for a sustainable win of your personal Right Size.

As you improve, brag and show off your **ScoreBook** and BB/Fatting Averages with friends and family. This is what I have found works best for me and how I do it. Find a way of **ScoreBooking** that is easiest for you!

FU Decision ("Fugly"): A Fat Ugly decision, like downing a Twinkie instead of grapes.

BB Decision ("BB"): A Body Beautiful decision, like eating an apple instead of a brownie.

Keeping Score with Your ScoreBook

If you have ever kept score in baseball or card games like bridge, you know scoring principles. The way Fat Warriors keep score is simple, and easier to learn and use.

Suggested Ideas & ScoreBooking Glossary

FU	Fugly--used for Fat decisions or Fat foods
BB	BB--used for good decisions
B	Breakfast
L	Lunch
D	Dinner
S	Snack
d	Drink--alcohol or sugar-based beverages
E	Exercise

Here are some decision examples that will show you how easy it is to keep score:

- **Foods you select**: For example, a brownie is an FU and an apple is a BB.
- **Portion sizes**: A portion size that is too large or too small is an FU, and a Right-Sized portion is a BB.
- **Bad decisions**: Starving or skipping a meal like breakfast is an FU.
- **Having a healthy breakfast**: Oatmeal, banana, whole-wheat toast and juice = BBs.
- **A not-so-healthy breakfast**: A jelly roll is an FU.
- **Daily exercise**: This is a BB, and an extra-long session might be two BBs.
- **No exercise**: Always an FU.
- **Indulging a Fat Ugly habit ("Fabit")**: For example, raiding the fridge at 11:00 p.m. is an FU.
- **Giving up a bad Fabit**: Not grazing on snacks while watching TV is a BB.
- **Having sex**: At least one BB, sometimes two. Remember, this should be fun!

First, prioritize a few key Fuglies and Fabits that you want to change. In fact, you may want to list your Fuglies and Fabits. Make these your priority decisions for starters.

ScoreBooking makes you more aware of big decisions, letting you wear smaller clothes.

Decisions Scoring, Not Food or Calories, Etc.

BB and FU decisions are what you will be measuring. You will not be measuring food, exercise, portions or calories. You may customize your decisions to what makes the most sense for you. My best example is that I used to have a ritual of snacking every night. Now any time I make the decision to skip this ritual Fabit, I reward myself with a BB in my ScoreBook. By doing this, those nocturnal calories and guilt do not lie in my stomach and weigh on my mind, disturbing my digestion and sleep. If I decide to have a late-night snack, it goes into my ScoreBook as a Fugly and lies with me all night long.

This means recording decisions like eating a large portion or more than one portion as an FU, and a properly sized healthy portion as a BB. **Eating a portion that's too small or nothing at all records as a Fugly, because deprivation is neither healthy nor sustainable.** Similarly, daily exercise is a BB, and no exercise is a Fugly. A movie tub of FatCorn is an FU, while diet soda may be a BB, depending on whether you believe in zero calorie sweeteners or not. Alcohol drinks (yes, even beer and wine) are Fuglies, so if you drink, cut it down. Each drink you skip is a BB. Each drink you have is an FU.

Say Yes to Nots

"Nots" can be BBs: not eating food after the evening meal, not snacking while watching TV, not eating high-calorie rich desserts, not eating high-fat foods, not pigging out at work, not downing bags of chips, and more.

You will become aware of your BBs and Fuglies and see that they reach much further than just food. **Daring to be aware and thinking about your decisions and consequences will help you make better decisions for your Right Size goal.**

Selecting an all-you-can-eat stuffet for dinner should qualify for two Fuglies just for deciding to enter, plus add more FUs for what you eat and huge portions. Stopping a Fabit, like eating at a stuffet or downing doughnuts at the office meeting, is a BB in itself. Not eating anything after 7:30 p.m. is an Oprah rule and is worth one BB, possibly two. These decisions are your call on scoring, depending on how bad your Fabit is or was.

You will occasionally make FU decisions, and starting out you may make many. Your goal will be to improve constantly until you make 10 or fewer Fuglies per month. ScoreBook them, be honest, record, and average. Feel good being aware and improving. Warriors theory is that if you make 10 or fewer FU decisions per month, you will naturally go from Fat Ugly to Body Beautiful.

If you do make your goal of ONLY 10 Fuglies per month, then you can convert them to BB decisions. The logic for the conversion from FUs to BBs is that you planned the 10 FUs and with discipline, you did not go over 10. At the end of the month, if there are 10 or less Fuglies, then convert and count them as BBs. It is the bonus for sticking with your plan and having the discipline to make it happen. However, it will take time to make this improvement because no one is perfect.

ScoreBooking and averaging decisions is key to your Right-Sizing victory. Anyone can do it. **You will understand why scoring and averaging is crucial to your self-motivation and discipline for winning your LGFG lifestyle.**

Real ScoreBook Examples of the Fat Warrior

I use the same abbreviations provided above in my ScoreBook: **B**=Breakfast, **L**=Lunch, **D**=Dinner, **S**=Snack, **E**=Exercise, **d**=drink. I also make small letter notations beside my Fuglies and BBs to help me remember what contributed to each decision. You may choose to do this, too, so you can see what led to your BB and Fatting Averages. You may want to develop your own scoring codes.

B: BB, BB (oatmeal with banana & berries, and whole-wheat toast)

E: BB (one BB for each 30 minutes of exercise)

S: BB-a (apple & raw almonds)

L: BB, FU (grilled chicken breast, and potato salad with mayonnaise)

D: BB, FU-d, FU-d (proper portion of grilled fish with two glasses of wine)

Your BB Average vs. Your Fatting Average

We know how important the batting average is to baseball players. The same importance applies to Fat Warriors performance. **Instead of a batting average, in Fat Warriors you will have a Body Beautiful Average ("BB Average") and a Fat Ugly Average ("Fatting Average").**

To calculate your **BB Average**, take your total number of BB decisions and divide by your total number of BB and FU decisions.

To calculate your **Fatting Average**, take your total number of FU decisions and divide by your total number of BB and FU decisions.

So for example, out of 10 decisions made this day, nine of them were Fat Ugly, and one was Body Beautiful.

➤   Nine FU decisions out of a total of 10 FU & BB decisions = Fatting Average of 900.

➤   One BB decision out of a total of 10 FU & BB decisions = BB Average of 100.

Keep in mind that the total of your Fatting Average + BB Average will always be 1,000 or 1.0.

Example: BB Average

➢   Seven BB decisions divided by 10 total BB and FU decisions equals a BB Average of 700 (7 BBs / 10 total decisions = .700).

Example: Fatting Average

➢   Three FU decisions divided by 10 total BB and FU decisions equals a Fatting Average of 300 (3 FUs / 10 total decisions = .300).

Remember, the sum of your BB Average and Fatting Average will always be 1000 or 1.0.

Great News!

If you are currently Fat Ugly, then your Fatting Average will be high and your BB Average will be low. The great news is that you only need to start making small improvements slowly to win more BBs and begin regaining your Right Size, complete with a healthy new lifestyle. **You will have grins instead of chins.**

You only need total focus on hitting more BBs and swinging at fewer Fuglies. At first, like learning to hit a ball, it will be difficult, but it will become easier because you will learn to be a better decision hitter. **Amazing but true, after a while it will be so easy that you will change and soon prefer the apple instead of the brownie.**

More Fun Examples of BB and Fatting Averages

Tally your FUs and BBs at the end of the day and end of the week, and calculate for Fatting Average and BB Average once a week. These averages will propel you to the best decisions and your best personal Right Size. It is a walk-off winner for you.

Pretend you have read the Fat Warriors book and you are now an experienced Fat Warrior. You have your eye on the BB decision ball and you record 100 decisions in one week--90 BBs and 10 FUs.

Again, for your **BB Average**, take your total number of BB decisions and divide them by your total number of BB and FU decisions:

➤ 90 BB decisions divided by 100 total BB and FU decisions equals a BB Average of 900 (90 BB / 100 total decisions = .900).

For your **Fatting Average**, take your total number of FU decisions and divide them by your total number of BB and FU decisions.

➤ 10 FU decisions divided by 100 total BB and FU decisions equals a Fatting Average of 100 (10 FUs / 100 total decisions = .100).

Your Fatting Average dropped from 900 to 100 and your BB Average rose from 100 to 900. See how recording and calculating your averages lets you track the dramatic improvement toward your Looking Good, Feeling Good lifestyle? ScoreBooking is the key to self-motivation and discipline to make your dream lifestyle become reality, permanently.

Pain in the Butt?
ScoreBooking should be painless and take no more than a couple of minutes a day. At the end of the day or at any time, write down your decisions for the day or the last few days. For example, once daily I record my scores in my ScoreBook. I do this at whatever time is most convenient. One evening I might take out my ScoreBook and record my decisions for yesterday and today. Sometimes I do it in the morning as I recall what decisions I made yesterday, but mostly I do it in the evening. **This 60-second investment in my Body Beautiful is well worth it.**

Think of It As YogaLight
In the morning, I mentally prepare for the BB and FU decisions I will face that day. I am consciously planning by practicing YogaLight. YogaLight is quick mental concentration for winning my Right-Sizing decisions by visualizing. I am ready as a Fat Warrior to begin to win the decisions of the day as I visualize and dream of my LGFG lifestyle.

It really becomes motivating fun when you start keeping your BB Average and Fatting Average. It is easy, quick, and will cause pride smiles as you improve.

Turn Up the Music, Step on the ScoreBooking Accelerator, and Enjoy the Drive

By ScoreBooking, soon you will be breaking Fabits and the pain of change is in your rear view mirror. The powerful benefits of ScoreBooking will make you stronger, happier, and more positive about yourself as you win back your Body Beautiful. Each BB decision will be a little badge of victory. You will eventually have strings of BBs, bringing feelings of achievement and lifestyle-changing victory.

Some say it works best to break ScoreBooking into small chunks, so do one month of ScoreBooking to experience it and see the progress it helps deliver. Your ScoreBook will be quite revealing of your Right-Sizing decisions and reveal your best Hot Bod. **You'll get an idea of how many Fabits you have, when they happen, and when you change them. Take one baby step, breaking one Fabit at a time, and commit to ScoreBooking for one month now!**

12

GREAT EXAMPLES OF FUGLIES AND BBs

Below are some great examples of Fuglies (Fat Ugly choices) and corresponding BBs (healthy food substitutions):

FUGLIES	BBs
Diet dominated by processed foods	Cook your own turkey or chicken. Buy lean meats and organic fruits & veggies.
Huge portions	Eat right-sized portions and practice The 20-Minute Rule to avoid over-eating.
Not eating breakfast	Eat the right foods early and often.
Sausage & hash browns breakfast	Substitute a colorful fruit plate.
Mega-sized fruity muffins	Just say No!
SuperSizeMyButt deluxe burger	Go with a grilled chicken salad with low or no-cal mayo.
Salad buffet with bleu cheese & dressing	Skip the oily, fatty dressing, go for a squeeze of lemon.
Peanut butter & jelly sandwich	Peanut butter on one piece of whole-wheat bread only (open-face style).
Snacking on chips and dips	Opt for healthy snacks (baked, not fried) plus fruits, veggies, raw almonds, etc.
Ice cream and sweet-tooth treats	Cut down on sugars and sweets.

FUGLIES	**BBs**
Milk shake	Try a fruit smoothie with fat-free milk.
Coffee shop Fat Dome with whipped cream	Regular coffee or tea without cream or with artificial sweetener.
Sugar-laden soft drink or fruit drinks loaded with sugar	Instead, drink diet soda, bottled water or tea.
Too much wine or beer	Cut down on alcoholic beverages.
Eating to stuffed fullness at restaurants	Share big meals at restaurants with a friend.
Eating too fast & shoveling food down	Chew each bite 10 times water between bites. before you swallow. Sip water between bites.
Couch potato TV watching with unconscious munching	Walking, jogging or biking can be done while TV-ing. Watch TV without eating.
Bedtime treats or raiding the fridge at night	Break that Fabit, no eating after dinner. Drink a cup of decaf hot tea or water with lemon.
No exercise.	Exercise, no matter how little. Try a walk or stretch after dinner.

List your Top 10 Fuglies and BBs on our website at www.FatWarriorsNation.com

Grocery Stores Are Stocked Full of BBs and Fuglies

Grocery shopping presents many decision opportunities when selecting foods to cart home. Score yourself one BB for the decision not to select predominantly FU foods, as well as for the decision to purchase BB foods. These are two big decisions, because **if FU foods are not selected and purchased, they can't be eaten at home to wear outside**.

Grocery carts filled with Fabits are called Grabits. Think first, before you grab. Go shopping with a list. If you use coupons, select ones for BBs. If you purchase BBs instead of Fuglies, you are stocking your home with healthy food that will make you look and feel great. You will also save money by not purchasing expensive junk food.

Rate Your Grocery Cart

Cart your future at the grocery store by rating the items in your grocery cart. What is important is that you are aware when you make an FU or BB decision at the grocery store. I do not count every item. Instead, I rate my grocery cart as a whole. So for example, I rated my cart as two FUs and six BBs with just a glance. Make it easy and quick. You do not have to count the 30 items purchased, but rather just use your judgment in scoring. Keep it simple and give yourself some credit for your great decisions!

Fat Warriors Rule:
Reduce your Fuglies to reduce your waistline.

Illuminate, Not Eliminate, All Fuglies

Illuminate your life with understanding and controlling Fuglies, but don't think you must completely eliminate them. Not making any FU decisions is not sustainable or realistic behavior toward living a full life. Your goal should never be to eliminate all Fuglies, but rather to gain a positive balance by constantly improving until you make BBs your dominant lifestyle. It is just reversing what made you Fat Ugly. **Your goal is to improve constantly one decision at a time, one day at a time, all the time.**

By decreasing your Fuglies and increasing your BBs, you will move slowly but naturally from Fat Ugly toward Body Beautiful. So cut out the junk and go for the alternatives instead. By keeping track of your Fatting Average and BB Average, you will be able to see progress in days won, weeks won, and months won. You will be heading toward sustainable behavior that can be permanent. Reaching your Right Size is obtainable. **Make your mantra: "I will rebound only in basketball."**

We expect you are occasionally going to make decisions to indulge in Fuglies. These indulgences will be in YOUR CONTROL AND A PART OF YOUR PLAN. Remember, it is in your control not to blow all your calories on a bulk meal, to add fitness and exercise to your lifestyle, to read labels, to go for lower-fat recipes and healthy snacks, and to resist extra helpings.

Fat Warriors do not ask you to give up anything except a dominating unhealthy lifestyle of Fat Ugly foods and inactivity.

Fabits Can Out-Eat Exercise Any Day, Every Day

The trickiest thing is portion size per serving = X calories. But who eats 10 potato chips or a quarter of a cookie? A fun way to measure a serving is by the number of miles of jogging it takes to burn it off. **Yes, a can of pop or beer should tell you about 1.5 miles, potato chips 3 miles, doughnut, or pastry 4-6 miles, etc.**

One mile of jogging burns off approximately 100 calories, depending on the jogger. **A piece of cake is no piece of cake when it becomes 5 miles of jogging.** What about cupcakes, pancakes and shortcakes? Any time you hear the word "cake," start running 5 miles immediately. Alfredo Sauce was not a name of a drunken sailor. Anything named Alfredo means jogging to avoid artery clogging. Fat Domes of whipped foams: run 7 miles. The extra-large size means run forever.

Now think about it: Would you run 4 miles to burn off a doughnut? If so, then eat it and run 4 miles to break even. Note that it takes jogging 5 miles to burn off love handles from an order of fries, 1 mile per beer.

You have to run many miles to out-eat big-out pizza. It is true you can have a couple of slices, but can you stop at 2, 3, or eating the entire thing? Eat the entire pizza for a free spare tire or run a marathon to burn it off.

The rule is to not out-eat your exercise. Exercise may help you gain energy and lose the tired feeling. You don't need to join an expensive gym or buy fancy equipment, unless you choose to. Start walking, bending, stretching, swimming, hiking, and biking whenever possible and encourage others to join you. Sign up for a 5K. Turn on the fitness channel and try a few workouts. The more time you spend exercising, the less time you will spend eating.

Once you start regularly exercising, you will change your mind and behind. You will start feeling great and re-energized, as opposed to being sluggishly depressed because you didn't.

Relentless on Your BBs

Maybe you can't make all of the BB decisions covered in this book, but you can make some of them! Then you will have momentum to make more, and that will reinforce positive behavior. **Keep your eye on your goal of Looking Good, Feeling Good and go to that mirror.** It takes one decision at a time, one day at a time, to reach your personal Right Size.

The more relentless you are about BBs and the more you visualize yourself making them, the more you will make. The reward is not taste, but looking and feeling healthier. BB decisions may be hard at first, but as you make them more often they will become easier and a comfortable part of your lifestyle.

Rule of Positive Decisions:
When I make a positive decision, I feel good.
The more I make, the better I feel.

Rule of Negative Decisions:
When I make a negative decision, I feel bad.
The more I make, the worse I feel.

Stand Up to Strawberry Shortcake

Maybe you are just a coward and afraid to stand up to strawberry shortcake. **What's really hard is standing up to all the traumas that you go through imprisoned by Fat Ugly.** If you think about it that way, you will find making BBs challenging, but worth the positive outcomes. Saying no to ice cream is much easier when you tack on a loss in love life, heart attack, stroke, or diabetes. Take on the battle. Show your War Face and growl. You will scare the ice cream back into the cone.

You may think that you will die when you first start making BB decisions, but not eating ice cream for a month will not kill you. Making FU decisions may be easy with instant taste gratification, but afterwards long-term depression sets in. Remember, you are at war with fat. The fact is that these fat decisions also kill many things, including people.

Eye on the Ball to Hit Your Right Size

In baseball and softball, coaches teach players that the art of hitting begins with keeping your eye on the ball. You just can't be a good hitter without keeping your eye on the ball.

To hit your Right Size, you must have your eye on the ball. That ball is **decisions!** It is not scales or calorie counting. Assuming you know the difference between a brownie and a banana, your eye must focus on the decision to go with the banana. If your eye focuses on scales and calorie counting, you will be thinking about the brownie and it will dominate your thoughts and find your mouth. You will see the brownie instead of the banana, the apple pie instead of the fresh apple, or the fried rice instead of the steamed veggies. You get the picture.

When you do not have your eye on the ball, you will not hit your Right Size. You will stay FU forever. To win your war, your thoughts must be on the decision to have the banana over the brownie, the 6-inch lean sub over the 12-inch five-meat sub, or a handful of nuts over the whole jar.

Remember: Eye on the decision ball, not scales or calories. War Face on. You know what is good and bad!

Mind Over Fatter

Decisions are from the mind, are provided by the harvest of your thoughts, and are 100 percent homegrown organic. You are directly responsible for your own decisions, and only you can make them. Your success has everything to do with what is inside of you. It all attributes to you, not diets, magical plans, or miracle pills. **It is within you, and you are a result of your self-empowerment. You alone have the power to make better decisions. This is the concept of Mind Over Fatter.** For once, you are in charge, in control, and you confidently know this is true.

13

STAND UP OR PORK UP

Law of Forever Fat: The pleasure of temporary taste is stronger than my will to make good decisions. Therefore, I will wear the temporary fat pleasure and live with the fat lifestyle of depression, embarrassment, and bad health forever.

FAT WARRIORS EXAMPLES OF PORK-ME-UP FABITS

PORK-UPS	WHERE	WHEN
Fridge-raiding for snacks	Home	Late night
Ice cream	Home	Until gone or dawn, whichever comes first
Texas-sized portions	Anywhere	Anytime
Potato chips, fries	Anywhere	Lunch, snack or dinner
No exercise	Nowhere	Never
Fataurants	All-you-can-eat stufferies	Anytime
Drive-throughs	Anywhere	Anytime

Pork-Me-Up Foods and Drinks

You, the reader, will write this chapter. List your top 20 pork-up behaviors plus foods and drinks. List where and when you get them and where they are readily, temptingly accessible. If you don't walk in mine fields, then you will not blow yourself up. It is important that you write this, as this will help you win your war against these builders of Fat Ugly and the depression they foster. You will then War Face them into former Fabits. Yea, it is another victory!

Your Top 20 Pork-Up Foods and Drinks

PORK-UPS	WHERE	WHEN
1.		
2.		
3.		
4.		
5.		
6.		
7.		
8.		
9.		
10.		

PORK-UPS	WHERE	WHEN
11.		
12.		
13.		
14.		
15.		
16.		
17.		
18.		
19.		
20.		

List Your Top 20 Pork-Up Foods and Drinks on our website at www.FatWarriorsNation.com

14

SELF-TALK BECOMES ACTION AND BELIEFS

Self-Talk: Atomic Fat Blaster

Your Self-Talk Is Always Right When it Comes to Your War on Fat

Your command center may be programmed to enjoy the pleasure of bigging out on Fuglies and oversized portions if you are currently FU. If you are programmed to attract Fat Ugly, your Self-Talk can deprogram and reprogram to attract Looking Good. **Your Self-Talk and imagery are always there for you to call on and utilize to your advantage. Self-Talk is free: no expensive plan, no contract, and no minute limit. Only one salesperson to deal with, and that is YOU!**

Your Self-Talk may tell you the pain is not great enough to give up those Fugly goodies. If so, you will eat them. Self-Talk may tell you that you can't win your war on fat. In that case, you are a doomed victim of Self-Talk and must resign as a Fat Warrior. Turn in your War Face and sit on the couch, grow wide hide, and watch until you are ready to fight for your personal Right Size.

Self-Talk may say the change in eating habits and lifestyle is worth the benefit of getting more attention from the opposite sex. **Self-Talk may convince you to make the BB decisions that will lead you to the front lines, from spectator to participating lifestyle.**

Self-Talk is the weapon of Fat Warriors that fat fears most. No spies in the world can tap into, control or hear Self-Talk. It is your unique and powerful weapon. People make fun of people talking to themselves, but Fat Warriors applaud Self-Talk. You Self-Talk the pounds right off your fat behind if you direct your decisions and thinking to looking and feeling your best. **As long as you keep talking to yourself and saying you can win, you are never defeated.** Self-Talk should be the best talk you have all day!

__Law of Override Depression__: Your body is the barometer of how you feel. If you look and feel Fat Ugly, that feeling will override to dominate your thoughts about yourself.

When you start Looking Good and Feeling Good (LGFG), that feeling will dominate your thoughts and beliefs. Your thoughts become your beliefs whether or not they are factual. What you believe you will achieve.

Beliefs Are True, Even if They Are Not

Whatever you believe is reality for you. If you believe it or perceive it to be true, then it is a fact to you even if it is not actually true in reality. For example, if you believe you will be Fat Ugly forever, you may think you will never be BB. However, if you believe you can achieve your best personal Right Size by making a few lifestyle changes, then you can beat FU.

Example: I grew up fishing with my dad, and one day a huge black snake came out from under the rock that I was sitting on and went between my legs. I screamed, could not breathe, and wet my pants. Other than that, it was a good fishing day. From that day on, however, I was afraid of snakes and, thus, going fishing. Snakes hang around water and some are poisonous, like the Water Moccasin. There are hundreds of snakes in the grass. You have heard the expression, "a snake in the grass." This is cowboy talk for a weasel of a person who is sneaky, like a snake slithering through the grass.

When I was in college, I lived with two guys in an apartment and was terrified of snakes. One roommate was a farmer's son; he neither liked snakes nor was afraid of them. The other roommate was a biology major who loved, hunted and kept caged snakes as pets. We were three different people. A snake in the room got three different reactions. My belief was that the snake would bite me, squeeze me to death, and then swallow me. The farmer thought the snake was just another animal. The biology major would be joyous: "Yea, another snake, let's party!" The snake itself was the same, but the three different beliefs caused three different sets of feelings and reactions that were true to each individual.

Scrutinize your beliefs and get them in concert to help you fight to become your personal Right Size. Shed any counterproductive Self-Talk that will stop you from controlling your weight. Your positive Self-Talk and thoughts will do the rest to have you eat healthier, lose weight, keep it off, and look and feel your best. **The fact is, you can decide on the apple over the brownie via Self-Talk and beliefs.**

Law of Attraction
The Law of Attraction is a theory that what you envision, think about, talk about and associate with becomes reality in time. It is like the movie "The Secret." What you visualize you will attract. Visualize healthy and you will attract healthy. Visualize driving your Best Bod and it will lead you to the Winner's Circle. Think about and visualize Looking Good, Feeling Good, and it will happen. Law of Attraction will help you battle fat.

Law of Fattraction
Just as the Law of Attraction says that what you think about will come to you, if you are distracted from your goal by constantly thinking about the pleasures of Fugly foods you will attract Fat Ugly. This is the Fat Warriors Law of *Fattraction*. Visualize fat and you will attract fat.

What you believe will be your truth and translate into your feelings and actions.

Believe to Achieve Mind Over Fatter
Lay your doubts aside and believe to achieve a Looking Good, Feeling Good lifestyle. It must be what you want most and you must visualize it. It must dominate your thoughts to empower BBs over Fuglies. Right Size with the power of Mind Over Fatter.

You will never give up because you have Pit-Bull mentality and are destined to win your war. You must have an absolute belief that you can win and will win. That becomes your only acceptable choice. Put your War Face on, war on, read on! Mind Over Fatter. **You can do it!**

15

FIGHT FAT OR FLIGHT FAT, BUTTS CAN'T HIDE

Emotional Plus Physical Pain Can Kick Fat Bully Butt

Fight or Flight

Fight or Flight is a law of nature. In a scary situation, you will either take flight and run or fight. Stress, overeating and little exercise can kick the body into fight or flight mode. However, running is not an option for Fat Ugly, so you must fight to win your personal Right Size and LGFG lifestyle.

Punch Your Fat Bullies

I learned as a kid that my enemy kid was the bully. He loved bullying me around, shoving and embarrassing me in front of my schoolmates. I was afraid of him, but too cowardly to do anything about it. Therefore, he pushed and shoved me around even more for added humiliation.

To make matters worse, I became the target of "wannabe bullies," and others started pushing me around, watching my tears flow and kids laugh. I did not know what self-esteem was at that time, but mine was gone and replaced by cowardice. I finally could not take it any longer and went to the toughest guy I knew that would certainly beat up the eight-year-old bullies: I went to my tough dad. I knew that he would have sympathy and beat up the bullies. I was wrong!

I told my dad about the bullies and my fear. He did not give me any sympathy. He told me that I was a coward and others bully cowards, it was that simple. Wow! That hurt as much as the bullying. Dad then added a little extra pain by telling me that as long as I let the bullies push me around and embarrass me, the more that would encourage them. A cycle of more pain. Where was the paternal love and sympathy? It was there, but placed with a lesson of stand up, get mad, and fight.

"OK, Dad, I am giving up the life of a coward and will stand up and fight. What do I do?" He said, "You plan. Pick the time and give him the sucker punch right on the nose." He showed me exactly how to throw the surprise sucker punch directly to the nose and follow with a one-two-plus-kick.

The bully came and bullied. When he glanced at the other kids laughing at me, I uncorked my first sucker punch right on his nose. His blood flowed, followed by his tears. Dad was right. I went from the coward to the one-punch kid. The bully and I did not become best friends, but he never got close to me again.

If you understand this story, you will understand that you must stand up to win your war on fat. Do not give into your Fat Bullies like SuperSizeMyButt meals, potato chips, apple pie, cheesecake, chocolates, or ice cream. Sucker punch them right on their noses.

Fat Bullies attack your positive lifestyle from their dark alleys.

Fat Bullies the Fat Warrior Turned into Lifestyle Changes

- **Ice Cream**: This Fat Bully hangs around dark alleys like the freezer and the Dairy Queen. **Sucker Punch**: Remove the ice cream from your freezer, replace with frozen fruits and stay clear of The Queen.
- **Potato Chips**: The dark alley is the pantry. **Sucker Punch**: Don't buy them at the store and you won't store them on your bod. Chip and dip only two times per month and eventually chip dip fever will almost disappear.
- **Cheeseburger and Fries at Fataurants**: The fast food drive-through window is the dark alley. **Sucker Punch**: Eat at home and have fast food only once a month. Substitute wheat bread and use fresh-cut potatoes to make baked fries.
- **All-you-can-eat Buffet for $9.95**: The pig trough stuffet is the dark alley. **Sucker Punch**: Don't go in.

- **MochaChocaLatte**: The dark alley is the coffee shop. **Sucker Punch**: Illuminate the dark alley with regular coffee or tea with artificial sweetener and creamed with skim milk. Coffee shops can have better choices.

List Your Top 10 Fat Bullies!

Name your Fat Bullies and record them in your ScoreBook. Once you have listed them, indicate how you will sucker punch them. Every morning as you brush your teeth, visualize your new, positive lifestyle, and plan your Fat Bully attacks.

Define the amount of pleasure time you receive from Fat Bullies and weigh that against the amount of pain you feel after consuming them. When you compare and see the lack of balance of pleasure to pain, it will make you ready to fight.

What are your Fat Bullies and sucker punches? List them on FatWarriorsNation.com and view others!

Commitment: One Week or Be Weak

During Pain Week, define all of the emotions the Fat Bullies inflict on you. Write them down, feel their inflicted pains and think about the hurt. How much do the Fat Bullies hurt you mentally, physically, and cost you? Think of the emotional cost, lifestyle cost, health cost, and financial cost. Fat Bullies are mean and tough and they love to inflict mental, monetary and physical pain on you. Their punches are Fat Ugly; they make you carry it and take your lunch money too.

Identify your Fat Bullies every day. You don't want to let any Fat Bully get away when you start delivering your powerful sucker punches, kicks, and elbows! War Face ON!

Fat Bullies Push Your Stomach Out and Around, Encasing You in Layers of Girth, Not Mirth

The pleasure time gained from Fat Bullies, balanced with the amount of emotional and physical pain they inflict is not balanced in favor of you feeling good about yourself. As an example, if you feel that your time ratio is 90 percent feeling bad from Fat Bullies and only 10 percent feeling good, then you may be motivated to sucker punch your Fat Bullies.

Fight one Fat Bully at a time with one BB at a time, one day at a time, and one week at a time. You will soon notice Fat Bullies leaving you alone and picking on other fat people. That is their role, to pick on helpless others and imprison them in layers of fat.

Each day you will fight Fat Bullies and make knockout decisions, either Fuglies or BBs. Track your decisions and averages in your ScoreBook each day, week and month. You will always strive for improvement with more BBs, fewer FUs, and never give up. You will win one BB at a time until you have won your personal Right Size.

Defeating one Fat Bully means a fight. Defeating many Fat Bullies means WAR. As a Fat Warrior, with your War Face and Combat Growl you will declare war on your Fat Bullies. You have the Fat Warriors Nation fighting on your team!

Win your battles, and then help your friends and family sucker punch their Fat Bullies. Bring them into the Fat Warriors Nation!

16

DETRACTORS AND DIVERTERS OF ACHIEVING YOUR PERSONAL RIGHT SIZE

Scales belong on fish.

Scales Are Not a Weapon of Fat Warriors

Scales belong on fish and not as a part of your BB lifestyle. Weighing is just not working--the professional yo-yo dieter will attest. Waddlers weigh more than Body Beautifuls and weigh themselves more often. Why?

Yes, with a scale you can see instant results for quick reinforcement. The problem with instant gratification and daily weight checks is that they are short-sighted and proven over the years to bring nothing but rebound weight gain and another cycle of miracle plans, pills and wheel meals.

Scale Distraction

You wake up and go to the scale to see if you have lost weight. You are happy if you lost weight, even though you have been down this road before and gained it back. Now you focus on scales and weight loss. That is sad, looking down constantly thinking of losing weight.

Instead of looking down at your scale, wake up, look up, and review yesterday's decisions in your ScoreBook and tallies for the week. Plan the positive decisions that you will make today. Approach the day with a Can-Do, "I am the decision-maker" mindset. **Wake up, put on your makeup, and get ready to go to war for your better life.**

As you go through your day, count the BB decisions that are leading toward a lifestyle change and a healthier, sexier bod. Count the FU decisions that are keeping you in fat depression. Focus on making decisions that will lead you to your personal Right Size. **Step off the scale and step up decisions scoring! Weigh in with BBs rather than a scale.**

Scale Tossing As a Sport and Being a Sport

Toss scales out as far as you can, you do not want them under your feet to distract you. We call this scale tossing. You may toss them in the trash or toss them to a neighbor, but toss them out! (At least into the closet for you to bring out once per month.) Keep it out of sight, out of mind.

Scale tossing can be fun when you toss a perfectly good scale to your neighbor. Then explain the Fat Warriors strategy behind scale tossing. Toss this paragraph around the neighborhood.

If your girth suggests birth,
you don't need a scale to see it.

Diet Distracters

One of the biggest distractions to permanent Right Sizing is the fad diet. **Just for fun, play the Diet Name Game. How many diets can you name that were *guaranteed* to lose the fat but fell flat?** Fad diets provide the happiness of quick, temporary weight loss that in turn provides the horrors of rebound weight gain depression. Some guarantees are designed based on the failure of most people to follow an unsustainable program. *"Come back and pay us more, and we will help you to temporary thin again!"*

Decisions Made You FU and Can Make You BB

When somebody asks how much weight you have lost, reply by saying, *"I don't know, but my Body Beautiful decisions percentage is up to 50 percent and I have made three permanent lifestyle changes. I am on the slowest weight loss program in the world, and we don't weigh in. I am the turtle of fat loss and I will beat the rabbit. I measure decisions and lifestyle changes, not pounds."*

When you rise to this level of commitment, you will understand why you do not want your scale to distract you.

Closet Scale Peepers and Calorie Counters

Some say the Fat Warrior actually is a closet scale peeper. Nobody is perfect. We won't dismiss or demote anybody from Fat Warriors for closet scale peeping monthly or calorie counting when necessary. Sometimes scales and calorie counting are useful or just fun when you are winning your fat war. The Fat Warrior admits to a monthly scale peep.

Notes

17

YOUR TOOLS TO BUILD YOUR BEST BOD

Self-Control Is the Muscle Up to Right-Size Moderation

Lifestyle Changes That Kick Fat's Ass: Commit to Rules You Will Follow

1. **No eating while TV-ing or playing video games.** You must go to the kitchen to snack. Stand-Snacking equals less fat-packing.
2. **Keep fat snacks out of range.** You cannot have them if they are not around.
3. **No snacks after eating your evening meal.** NONE, but if you absolutely must have a late-night snack, eat an apple or orange, celery or carrots.
4. **Have one of your favorite Fuglies no more than once per week.** Yes, French fries once, or ice cream once, or cake once (not the whole cake), in a moderate portion size. Like most, you will not miss them after time.
5. **If you have a sandwich, make it open-face style to cut your intake of bread in half.** On multigrain, not white bread, of course.
6. **Reduce weekly pizza night to monthly pizza night. Cut number of slices eaten** to cut inches off your belly over the year. Skip the sausage and pepperoni and go for the green peppers and mushroom toppings instead. Better yet, make your own pizza with fresh tomatoes and low-fat cheese.
7. **Drink lots of water.** Candy will grow *on* your hip. Instead, carry a water bottle and *be* hip. A hand holding a bottle of water cannot hold a candy bar.

8. **Practice The 20-Minute Rule:** Don't eat until stuffed--stop when comfortable, wait 20 minutes, drink some water, and then see if you still want more. You probably won't, and the pain of Must Have More is soon eliminated, as are hundreds of calories and the bloated after-hogging feeling that always gets you down.

9. **Go nuts!** Keep apples and natural snacks like raw almonds in your car or bag for a great healthy snack, especially when going for a walk. This kills fat snacks.

10. **Eat healthy at home more often.** Food can be prepared quickly with low-fat recipes, which are healthier and less expensive than Fataurants.

11. **You must have physical activity.** You can dance, walk, garden, but MOVE. Just start moving and grooving.

12. **Don't cheat & don't hide.** Be honest with your friends, family, and most of all yourself. You are making good choices. Brag, don't hide sweet treats and Cheat-Eat.

13. **Chew your food.** Chew each bite 10 times before swallowing; savor and enjoy the taste before taking the next bite.

14. **Slow down your eating and use good manners.** Shoveling food in your mouth at record speed makes it less enjoyable to eat. Your family and friends at the table will view your rapidly paced eating as FUGLY.

What Lifestyle Changes Do *YOU* Need to Make?

An experienced nurse practitioner told me that she believes obesity is to the point of being obscene, and these people desperately need help. She has seen many obese patients who have tried diets and had short-term fixes, when they really needed to make long-term lifestyle changes for lasting results. Doctors agree with the premise that losing fat requires making the right food choices coupled with physical activity. Beautiful people look, and in general are, happy with their lives and bods. **Few of us are after the perfect model-thin figure, but rather the best personal Right Size that we can be to enjoy a happy, healthy lifestyle.**

For Right Sizing to be permanent, it must come as a *lifestyle* change. That change must be permanent for fat to stay off. It can't be the result of temporary behavior or it will only keep Fat Ugly away temporarily and keep it coming back with a vengeance.

Think of other decisions you have made that finally led to lifestyle changes, such as stopping or reducing smoking, drinking, caffeine usage, and other routines. For me, I was able to change 25 years of smoking to a lifestyle of nonsmoking.

I would not think about having a cigarette now. Foods, like the cigarettes, that no longer control me are ice cream, candy bars, doughnuts, pastries, pizza, and the beloved cheeseburger basket with drippy, greasy, wonderful-tasting, fat-laden, salt-absorbing, ass-building French fries. I occasionally have a basket, but find that happening less and less as I lose my taste for them just like cigarettes. I no longer have any pains from avoiding Fabits, because my lifestyle changed and the pains of not indulging have long since disappeared.

Focus on Right Sizing With the Power of Mind Over Fatter

Focus on making more BBs and visualize the rewards. When you focus, you can put on your War Face and be a decision-making, Fat Ugly-fighting machine. **Don't focus on losing pounds or you may lose your true focus. Your full focus and power of your mind must be on making decisions to attain and maintain your best personal Right Size, coupled with a Looking Good, Feeling Good lifestyle. Mind Over Fatter.**

Nothing Stops Passion Energy

Desire and dreams will give you passion energy. **Nothing stops passion energy. Passion energy is a choice, you can have it flow or you can TV it.** You may feel tired, a great excuse for TV, and forget the walk, but taking the walk or exercising when tired will likely cause a decrease in sluggishness and a reawakening in energy.

There is a difference between thinking you are tired and having no energy and actually being physically exhausted. Most of the time there is reserve energy in the tank. Push yourself. If you mentally call on it, you may well have energy to burn fat and feel much better after exercising. After exercise, you will be more relaxed, euphoric, and sleep well. **You're feeling good and on your way to winning your war on fat!**

Energy is easy when everything is fine. It's when things are tough and you are down on the canvas that you need to summon it up from the fiber of your being. The tough get going; it's there, bring it up. Use your War Face. Energy keeps things in motion. By keeping things in motion, you will have the momentum and energy to make BB decisions. **You will learn to yearn to burn.**

A running mate made me walk after dinner when I was tired and wanted to watch TV. She encouraged me to "just walk for 10 minutes." Well, that little walk woke my energy cells up and it became easy to do an enjoyable 20 minutes' walk with a friend after meals. I counted it as exercise and a BB decision, or 5-7 BBs per week. It will make a big difference over the long span of a year, or should I say *walk a short time for a long time of Looking Good, Feeling Good.*

A vulgar four-letter word that Fat Uglies hate:
MOVE

Exercise
The four-letter word that causes SWEAT? It is MOVE. You must have physical activity. You can dance, walk, garden, do yoga, Pilates, but MOVE! Whatever it takes, just do it!

How much do you exercise now? If your only exercise is getting up from the chair to go to the fridge, get moving. Eating right is the most important component to Looking Good, Feeling Good and having a Hot Bod.

Exercise is the best ally and a major Fat Warriors weapon when combined with eating right. Fat Warriors do not diet, but rather make good decisions, eat right, and exercise.

The right amount of the right things at the right time, along with exercise, is the treasure map to your personal Right Size.

Eating "Naked" food is healthy and you will acquire a taste for it. We call any food that is not wearing unhealthy salt, fats and bad stuff, "Naked" food.

Eat Naked!
Chemical-free food is best for you. **Eat fresh, natural, and organic foods.** Grow your own garden-fresh foods. Of course,

you can also try actually Eating *Naked* and you will see your bod results immediately as you swallow and wallow. You will eat less, and better, when you eat naked. P.S. Do not do this at a restaurant or at the church social. Eating Naked is usually done in private or with your best friend.

Imagine and Visualize Your Goals

Before a batter hits a home run, he has already thought about it and visualized it. It is not about the home run, it is about the crowd cheering, the girls, running for four bases, teammates patting him on the back, and helping win the game. The home run made many wonderful things happen.

Before a woman becomes an executive, she has already pictured it and then planned to make it happen. She has visualized the promotions, personal satisfaction, accolades from friends, money, and other benefits to her life.

I visualized writing this book and readers benefiting from it. **You must visualize your goals first before you can achieve them.**

Imagine Attaining the Steamy Dreamy Figure You Desire

Imagine being the ultimate fat-fighting machine. See yourself turning heads with your beautiful figure and making men dream. Men, picture you are handsome, looking good, and doing abs commercials. Picture it, think it, and you will get it. Law of Attraction is again working for you. When you see yourself as **Smoking Sexy Hot**, you are ready for the next visualization. Okay, the Fat Warrior has gone extreme on caffeine, but you get the idea. It's fairly simple: Think and picture good thoughts and you will attain them.

Fat food is the credit card that brings the Fat Ugly debt: Eat me now and pay for me later. I will show up on your bod at month's end.

Instant Gratification Control

People make impulse decisions to purchase themselves into debt. They also make impulse decisions with food. When this occurs, step back and think about the ramifications of the decision. How will it make you feel for the rest of the day when you wear it? Is it worth it? Use your Self-Talk to talk yourself out of making that bad FU decision.

Scales Steal the Moment--Mirrors & Buckles Tell Your Story

One of the best fat-fighting tools ever is the mirror. The mirror diagnosis tells the story of time, of days, weeks, years, and life. The scale is in the now, but the mirror shows the result of many decisions from yesterdays. **The mirror shows the dramatic effects from your past decisions.** What you decide to do today will at some point affect the mirror and the belt buckle diagnosis of the future.

The mirror takes an oath before it can become your mirror. The mirror oath is to never lie, but deliver you the truth. Therefore, you trust a mirror to show you the truth.

You can't fool the mirror, your belt buckle or your clothes.

The Mirror Knows and so Do Your Clothes

Your clothes also take the truth pledge, and they will camouflage but not lie. Your clothes show and make you feel the truth from yesterday's decisions. Clothes will punish you by first fitting you snug, and then too tight. Then they will choke you into buying at the big size store and dressing black as Fat Ugly returns.

First thing in the morning, go to the mirror and look at yourself. Put on your War Face and growl. Mirror, mirror, on the wall, who's the Best Bod of them all? Does Fat Ugly now cover the once beautiful prince or princess? Never fear. You will free yourself from the fat that imprisons your natural good-looking bod. Imagine the Body Beautiful you can have. Focus on the BB decisions needed to achieve it and win your war on FU!

Carry a Picture of You Fat and Looking Good

Carry a picture of yourself when you were BB or close to it. Look at it when you are tempted to make a Fugly decision. Better yet, carry a split photo--one side before, and one side fatter. Now, do you still want that innocent-looking cookie? You must weigh the good taste and five minutes of eating pleasure of the cookie against the pain of being fat 24-7. You must sing the song "Forever Fat."

Okay, there is no such song, but you can sing it anyway. You decide which you want and what is best for you. **Body Beautiful dream. Dream it, think it, and have it. That is the Law of Attraction.**

Saboteurs Are Terrorists and Should Be Dumped

Naysayers don't do, can't do, and they discourage doers. They are perverts and purveyors of destroying the discipline and will to succeed. Naysayers provide excuses, and they are terrorists trying to make you feel that it is okay to blow your body up to huge size. Saboteurs sabotage the fight out of people around them and perpetuate the comfort of failure by discouraging the possibilities of success. Just stay away from them and tell them they have too much negative karma for Fat Warriors. Show them your War Face, growl, and tell them you are a winner. **Like a bad tire, change them for a positive "Can-Do" team of friends.**

Support Groups or Support Hose

Connect to positive support groups that will help you become Fat Warriors. Examples:

- Seek out role models instead of dough models: mother, father, siblings, friends--anybody that will fight Fat Ugly
- Let positive people influence your lifestyle decisions
- Get a personal trainer, coach or friend to help you
- Join meetings or clubs of Can-Do people
- Don't hang with Fuglies that perpetuate eating FU
- Do hang with Healthies and BBs, and you will be on your way to trimming your trouble zones

Be Determined, Never Give Up

If you fall off the momentum wagon, figure out why and fight back so that falling off happens less and less over time. **Falling off the momentum wagon is a part of the process, so use your War Face, get back on, and ride.**

Example: When you lose your focus and order a SuperSizeMyButt meal, the next time you are tempted pull out your ScoreBook, put on your War Face, and give a quiet Combat Growl. Use your powers of Mind Over Fatter. You will probably not order it and instead go for the turkey sandwich on whole-wheat toast with lettuce and tomato, hold the mayo.

It is almost impossible to order a SuperSizeMyButt after giving a Combat Growl while wielding your Fat Warriors

ScoreBook. In a few minutes, you will feel the joy of your winning decision and not the depression of wearing the Fuglies all day. Happiness will prevail and unveil more BBs in your ScoreBook.

Never, ever quit and you will never be defeated. Always try to win one more BB decision, one decision at a time, until lifestyle change happens, leading you to belt-buckling victory.

18

HEALTH FOOD STORES
STORE HEALTH TREASURES

Who You Gonna Call? Fat Busters!

When you have a question about nutrition or supplements, who you gonna call? You will find a treasure of products, knowledge and friendly people at a health food and supplement store who will help you win your Best Bod, mind and spirit.

A super bod and mind begins with super decisions. One great decision is to walk into a health food and supplement store. Walk in and the staff will make you feel welcome. **Retailers of natural products understand and are willing to help people who are trying to improve their bodies, minds and spirits.** Fat Warriors know that there is a health food store just a jog or walk away.

Fat Warriors believe that more Americans are actively participating in the connection between good foods, natural supplements, weight, health, and happiness. More people than ever before are trading heavily processed foods for a selection of natural or organic foods and supplements.

Big Treasure in People

The greatest asset in the health food store is the team serving you. Talk to them, ask them, and embrace their knowledge and expertise. There are good and bad people in every profession except politics, and health food stores are no different. So you decide on your comfort level with the store and staff. You may then decide to buy or fly. Most stores tend to have great people on staff who are intent on helping you accomplish your goals.

Variety of Items Sold

Health food stores stock treasures of healthy foods, supplements, books, and other items. Example: The health food store staff may suggest that you steer clear of chemicals, preservatives, artificial dyes, or sweeteners that may not be included in many of the products they carry. Specialized foods are also available, like gluten-free foods. If they don't have something you want, they will likely order it. They love to make customers happy!

Mystery Novels vs. Team Knowledge

Reading labels is sometimes like reading a mystery novel. Like most, you may not be able to figure out what is good and what is evil for your bod, mind, and spirit. Health food stores are generally staffed with a team of knowledgeable people willing to help customers decipher labels and share their insights.

Health food store employees are usually upbeat and you will not wonder why. They tend to practice what they preach and sell. Most of the owners and staff got into the health food business because it is one of their passions. **Natural products retailers help their customers with decisions for a happier, healthier lifestyle. In the end, you decide. The End.**

19

WHY YOUR HOUSE HOUSES YOUR FUTURE BOD

_Reversal of Taste Rule__: Some good foods will not taste as good as fat foods at first, but the longer you eat healthy, the more you acquire a taste for healthy foods. The great news is that your taste buds will eventually lose their zest for the intense taste of fat foods._

Most good foods taste good and make you feel even better. Good foods promote health and happiness; bad foods promote high blood pressure, diabetes, low self-esteem, sad clothes, and other bad things. What is your choice for life?

Never Fill Grocery Carts With Groceries!

Check in for life or check out of life at the grocery store check stand. The items going down the conveyor belt to the cashier are not groceries! Yes, they look like groceries, and they charge you for them as groceries and people call them groceries, but they are not groceries. **Grocery carts are filled with _decisions_ that look and taste like groceries**.

If you decide to buy ice cream, whipped cream, sugar cereals, potato chips, and candy disguised as food, they are all your decisions to make you Fat Ugly. Put FU decisions in your grocery cart to cart home for growing your gigantic figure. Put BB decisions in the cart to dance home and embrace your Looking Good figure of tomorrow. Which do you choose?

Your Grocery Cart Is the Predictor of Your Future Looks and Feelings

Your grocery cart outweighs your scale with impact on your Right Size. **Look at your grocery cart instead of your scale.** Grocery cart decisions eat scales for breakfast and munch on calorie counters. Do you fill your cart with Fuglies or BBs? Your scale's bod impact score is zero, but your grocery cart scores dramatic bod effects.

What is on the checkout conveyor belt is conveying your future Body Beautiful, or belting out your waistline. What you see in the grocery cart is the future story of your FU or BB bod.

Packaged Food May Mean Packaged Fatness

Packages do not grow on trees, and farmers are not harvesting fields of boxes and packages. If food comes in a box or package, there is a good chance it is processed food, which may make your packaging fatter. Be aware. Fresh foods make you fresher. If Mother Nature grew them, then she meant you to look good wearing them. Cupcakes do not grow in fields, so put the packaged fat stuff back now.

Cart Peeping Can Be Fun *and* Legal

People are checking out your big-out grocery selections or your healthy foods. A good nutritionist could probably look at a grocery cart and guess the bod style of the owner. Look at grocery carts and then look at their owners. Watch the heavyweight shoppers and then look into their carts. Watch the BBs and look into their carts. **Cart peeping can be fun and a learning experience.** Play the game, peek at the cart, and guess the weight of the cart pusher. The closest wins an apple.

ScoreBook your grocery cart. Your action plan might start by making a list before you go and sticking with it. For a better score keep score, record, and compare your grocery cart Fuglies and BBs week to week for six months. You win the battle of the grocery cart and your belt-buckling victory is in sight.

Home Houses Grocery Cart Decisions

What is in your grocery cart goes into your house, then your mouth, and then you wear it. **The grocery cart tells the story of whether you live to eat or eat to live.** What you put in the cart dictates where you go to buy your clothes, what you look like, feel like, and your health.

You have stocked your home with what you look like. If you hide foods to fool anybody, you will only be fooling the fool and hurting yourself. So get it out in the open for you and everyone to see your selections. You will be proud to display good food that will help you look good.

Items in Your Pantry You Will Wear

Take a picture of your pantry. **Picture what you see in the pantry or fridge is what you will see in the mirror.** Do you see the cookies and potato chips in your mirror staring back at you? Potato chips advertise that you can't eat just one--are they suggesting that you pig out on them? All chips chip away at your willpower, so don't eat any and eventually avoid the pain of wanting them. Chips taste good, and even better with dip. Chips and dips help support your favorite weight loss programs. I was addicted to chipping and now I limit them or French fries to two times per month.

Stove, Table and Plate Reality Show

The **stove** cooks the food of fat bods and Hot Bods alike. It makes no judgment.

The **table** is a picture of the future family figures. Figure that and make better decisions.

The **plate** holds your FU or BB decisions before they move into and onto your bod. Plates stacked high with food, filled to the brim ruin trim. The Fat Warrior does not advocate wasting food, so take small portions. If you clean your plate, remember what goes on the plate in excess also goes on your butt in excess.

Hidden Treasures Are Visible on Your Waistline

Is your nightstand or purse loaded with munchies, chocolate, candy, or other pork-up treats? I love it when people say, "Well, it is dark chocolate and that is good for me." It may be if you are at the Hot Bod stage. However, calories hide in the dark and you can't see them, even in dark chocolate.

What fat food hides in your house that is standing in your way of winning your Best Bod?

The Living Room Is the Killing Room

The living room may be killing your bod if you couch potato it and chip dip while watching TV. The TV in the living room can be a death trap, baited with the opportunity to TV snack and die prematurely. Is this exaggerated? Maybe.

TV can be a great form of entertainment. It can also be an unhealthy form of "lay" entertainment as you watch and sit to be unfit. Too much TV promotes sitting, snacking, and flabby "grandma arms," with little exercise found in chip dipping. TV, along with video games, may be surrounding your body with that depressing Fat Ugly look.

I like my TV, but I also like BB. If you have time to TV pork up, you also have time to walk, run, or bike. Watch TV, but do so with good judgment and no snacking and fat packing during viewing. Learn to enjoy TV snack free!

Lose weight while watching TV.
Make TV snack free!

20

PIG OUT ON SUCCESS, NOT ON FAT

Instead of Fuglies, Take a Bite Out of Life.

Fattest Myths

- **I exercised, so I can have that doughnut, chocolate chip cookie or just eat like a hogger.** *If you do this, you will out-eat your exercise, negating any benefit.*
- **Jogging and going to the gym alone will make me thin.** *No, you must also eat right.*
- **Ice cream, cakes, and desserts make me fat.** *Wrong, <u>eating</u> them makes you fat.*
- **McDonald's made me fat, the fast food industry made me fat, trans fats made me fat.** *They did not hold a gun to your spoon and fork!*
- **My genes made me fat.** Many people believe this and it may be true for some. *However, genes usually do not put the pie in your pie hole.*
- **My clothes make me look fat.** *Wrong, it is YOU in your clothes that makes you look fat.*
- **Wearing black makes me look thin.** *If you are fat, wearing black just makes you look fat in black.*
- **Horizontal stripes make me look fat.** *If you are Fat Ugly, don't blame the stripes. (However, stripes on fatties do make them look like fat prisoners or a chubby New York Yankee.)*
- **If I wear a jacket, I can hide the love handles.** *Yes, but you must take it off sometime, surprise! Love handles are fat rings that are moving toward fat saddles.*

- **BBQ ribs are good!** *No, the poured sugar BBQ syrup sauce loaded with lots of calories is good.*
- **Grilled chicken salad loaded with Fat Ugly dressing is a Body Beautiful decision.** *Many dressings are loaded with fat calories and undo any good from eating the salad. Select the right dressing for a BB.*
- **"This food is better than sex."** *Only means that you have not had good sex.*

__Rule of Time & Taste__: "If it tastes good, then I must have one or treat myself to one." In a matter of minutes, the good taste is gone and the bad feelings linger, as does the fat forever. You wear and carry what you eat. For minutes fat foods taste real good, but make you feel bad for hours.

Slopping the Hogs, All-You-Can-Eat Trough

My Grandpa, a Kansas farmer, called feeding the pigs "slopping the hogs." The pig has no choice but to eat the slop, get fat, and be butchered. This slop is a concoction made to pork up the pigs before slaughter. In essence, the pig gets the slop at the trough and porks up just like people at Fataurants ordering SuperSizeMyButt meal portions.

The hogs love the taste of the slop and can't wait to eat it to the fullest. Is this how you feel? Pigs do not know that porking up leads them to slaughter. The faster they pork up, the sooner they die. **Is there any correlation to what the slop is and what some humans eat to the max?** Wild boars are lean, mean, fighting pigs and eat no slop. What can we learn from the wild boar and the farmer's pig?

Treat and Eat Myth

"I ran six miles, so I can eat this pizza, and a lot of it. I think I will put a big slice in each paw so that I can just cram it on my body and watch the fat break out." We call this treat and eat. You did a good thing but negated it with a bad choice. Forget the six-mile run, just tape a pizza box on your butt and walk around the off and show it off.

"I ate a salad yesterday, so for lunch today I will treat myself to this SuperSizeMyButt Fat Ugly meal with sugar-laden Joke Coke."

Use both paws and shovel it all down as fast as you can. Be sure to put a generous helping of ketchup on it, or just squirt the ketchup directly into your mouth, followed by tossing the salt packets on your tongue. Drink the creamy, thick malt so fast it gives you brain freeze.

"I took a walk today, so I would like to have some macaroni and cheese for a snack later. Tomorrow I will have a creamy casserole and some coconut cream pie."

Order your Fuglies this way: "May I have the brownie ice cream with fudge and nuts on the top, and 24 hours of follow-up depression on the side? And could you also bring me a side of new belt, as I am having trouble breathing in this one."

You get the idea of the Treat and Eat Myth.

Pig Out on Success

Pigging out on success is one of the best things you can do for Right Sizing. Think positive and pig out on celebrations of BB decisions and lifestyle changes. This is a most critical step in Right Sizing!

Pig-Out Positive Examples

* Celebrate even small positive decisions, such as choosing whole grain breads instead of white bread
* Cheer for yourself when you cart home a Right-Sizing grocery cart
* Reduce processed products--Eat Naked food without chemicals
* Pat yourself on the back when you reduce or limit Fabits (like eating after 7:30 p.m. or late-night fridge raids)
* Hang out with more BB people and less FUs
* Give yourself a prize when you reduce a belt buckle hole
* Visualize positive images of your bod, love life, job, and health

Notes

21

PARADIGM SHIFT WILL SHIFT YOUR FAT GONE

Fat Uglies Live to Eat, but Body Beautifuls Eat to Live.

If You Eat to Live, Most of Your Life and Time Will Be Directed at Having Fun and Owning Your Desires

We base this theory on the fact that you spend a total of about one hour a day actually engaging the mouth in eating. Now, oinkers may spend more time than that, but the dilemma exists. **This means you counteract one hour of fun eating tasty pleasures by 23 hours of feeling embarrassed, bloated, ugly, fat, sluggish, tired, and weak.** You do the math, and you may want to fight back. Be a Fat Warrior and enjoy the 23 hours.

Treat or Retreat?

Body Beautifuls believe in the paradigm of eating to live. They do not believe in gorging themselves with all the tasty morsels that come their way. They deliberately select when to treat and when to retreat. They live for the 23 hours of the day when they own Looking Good. The mirror is their friend, and they make friends more easily with the opposite sex. **You don't have to be a rocket scientist to figure the math of 23 hours vs. 1 hour.**

It is a small price to pay to change your paradigm from living to eat to eating to live. Think about it: enjoying minutes of taste pleasure vs. hours and days of Looking Good, Feeling Good, getting the girl or guy, getting the job, and getting your smile back.

Weigh That Thought

Does your Fat Ugly outweigh a lifestyle of Looking Good, Feeling Good? That is why you are now FU. Only when a paradigm shift occurs and Looking Good, Feeling Good becomes more important than your desire to gorge yourself will you arm to achieve the goal of your personal Right Size.

Body Beautiful people have a fun life before, during, and after food! **The astonishing thing is that BBs probably enjoy good food more than hoggers enjoy Fugly foods.** Fat Uglies can learn to like fruits, vegetables, lean meats, and less fattening foods. Body Beautifuls like them, and so will you if you try. You will find that some BBs eat things with weird names like tofu, but they also eat beef and everything else in moderation, which tends to moderate over health and happiness. **Sprinkle moderation on anything and it becomes better.**

Celebrate if you start hanging around with BB people, as you will pick up some of their healthy habits.

Make the paradigm shift to shift your fat gone for good!

22

FOOD FOR THOUGHT

Large Portion Rule: *Eating large portions at any time makes the stomach full, but your brain may not get the message until 20 minutes later. This gives you time to stuff the stomach uncomfortably full. Loosen that belt, unbutton those jeans. If it curves out, then you will fill out. If you eat thin, the stomach stays in.*

Small Plate Rule: *Big Plate means more taste but added feelings of stuffiness. Small Plate means a comfortably full, flat stomach, and Body Beautiful pride. The flat stomach lasts. The enjoyment of a stuffed, fat stomach is over quickly and turns to sluggish depression. It is your choice.*
Go happy, go BB, go Right Size.

The 20-Minute Rule: Impacting/Enhancing Love Life

After I made fun of Chicago Cubs Manager Lou Piniella's Santa Claus belly, Cutie let me know that I had grown the same Piniella Belly (complete with wrap-around stomach). That was more than I could stomach.

My ego shock set in with a dose of belt-tightening embarrassment. I did not realize I had gotten that fat because I was jogging four times per week. The fact was that **I was out-eating my exercise**, and my treats were defeating the miles that I was jogging.

When I had my first meal served by Cutie, I almost fell off my chair. First thing wrong, she served the meal on little plates, but that was not the topper. **I was used to cowboy-sized plates of piled-high food that was almost spilling over.**

99

When she brought out the smaller plate, it seemed against the Man Code and wrong. However, making it even more disheartening was that I could actually see plate between the foods. She did not pile the food high and actually left separation between foods. Forget about overflowing!

I pointed out to Cutie that I could not only see plate, but also the pattern of the entire Dutch windmill. This was wasting precious food space for art. She agreed that the windmill was exposed, but told me to just enjoy the food and the portion. Whoa. Cowboy cooking does not recognize the word *portion*. We use words like *piled* or *stacked* and *filled to the brim*. You *pile* but you do not *portion*.

Therefore, I did the smart, manly and polite thing and just called for seconds. That'll fix Cutie. Whoops, wrong. She told me that I would receive my seconds in *20 minutes*. But seconds should be served in seconds, not *minutes*. Since the seconds were only seconds away in the kitchen, why the 20 minutes?

Understanding my confusion, she said it was not kitchen travel time, but **The 20-Minute Rule.** If I would wait 20 minutes, then I might experience a phenomenon known as "You are full and don't need seconds to sprout your Piniella Belly." I could not believe it, but after 20 minutes I was fully food satisfied without eating more to extreme fullness. I checked my Piniella Belly and decided to smaller size it by not having seconds. I am now a disciple of The 20-Minute Rule.

The 20-Minute Rule will result in smaller portions and will produce a thinner you and Lou. The thinner me will produce a better love life as Cutie explained to me. Cutie put down the plates and we agreed that some things don't need The 20-Minute Rule.

The Orange Potato Chips Mystery

It is the Code of the West that a cowboy must have potato chips with a sandwich. Just like ham and beans, peanut butter and jelly, and salt and pepper go hand in hand, salty, crunchy, fatty potato chips must accompany a sandwich or it is just not complete.

You might say that a sandwich with chips is almost spiritual. A sandwich must have two slices of bread and salted potato chips to be in harmony with the planets and universe. Face it, an open-face sandwich is not really a sandwich, but rather a halfwich.

Cutie invited me to a private lunch picnic. I questioned her on the absence of the sandwich duet, and then I saw the wonderful sandwich and called for the potato chips. She pulled a plastic bag from the cooler and handed it to me saying, "Here are your potato chips."

I looked at the bag and quickly noticed that the chips were orange, and there is no orange in potato chips. In fact, I said they looked a lot like *sliced carrots*. Does that mean Lou Piniella Belly or orange potato chips? Lou Piniella Belly and a waistline that shakes like jelly. It was one of my lifestyle changes--sandwiches without potato chips. I have since lost my Lou Piniella Belly, gained a new chip ritual and love them. I also love Lou, but he needs to talk to Cutie.

Thanks, Lou, for the inspiration, and now win a World Series for the Cubs and you will be our hero. Call me if you need help with the belly or the Cubs. I have a lot of managerial experience in Little League.

Fish Eating

Cutie has tried to get me to eat more fish, but has not gotten this beef-eating cowboy to adopt that lifestyle change. Cheetahs are the fastest, leanest, and best-respected warriors in the animal kingdom. Cheetahs and lions eat only red, raw meat, roar, and have never been seen dining in a sushi bar.

If it does not moo, oink or cluck, I do not eat it. If an animal does not speak, I do not eat. That is my rule, and a rule shunned by some of our finest in the Fat Warriors Army.

I am the Fat Warrior and have my War Face on when it comes to eating fish. However, for the sake of other Fat Warriors, I understand that **fish is an extremely healthy food--a great source of protein, vitamins, and nutrients--and should be a regular part of weekly meals.**

Choose fish that are good for you such as wild salmon, rainbow trout, and albacore tuna. Bake, grill, or broil it, add some seasoning and lemon, serve with salad, baked potato, and fresh fruit, and you've got a million-dollar meal without a million calories!

I must confess that after starting to write this book, I have actually begun to acquire a taste for fish. What will be next, tofu?

Veg Out

I don't understand vegetarians. Once again, I never saw a lion vegetarian or lioness vegan, but some of our best Fat Warriors are vegetarians and vegans. Vegetables are great for you and they probably would give lions needed antioxidants. However, the tigers would laugh at lions eating broccoli. I think elephants and hippos are vegetarians. Sharks don't eat vegetables and pretty much eat meat or fish. I know tiger sharks eat worms, but I am not sure if a worm is meat or vegetable. I think worms belong to the food group called bait. You have heard of the term "bait and switch." I think sharks would eat a steer if the steer would swim under water in the ocean. Sometimes the Fat Warrior has too much coffee and spills some nonsense into his writing. Do you sense that at times?

Plan meals that make vegging out good for you and fun. For example: If you love pasta, add steamed veggies and meatless meatballs made with soy instead of ground beef for protein. Try a healthy whole-wheat wrap stuffed with green peppers, shredded lettuce, tomato, mushrooms, lean turkey or ham, and a little low-fat shredded cheese.

Sugar-Coat *This!*

Friends should not talk about three things. You will only infuriate and agitate, but will never change minds. These areas are politics, religion, and artificial sweeteners. Cutie hates artificial sweeteners, and makes me wash my hands after handling the packets. Therefore, at great risk of being proven wrong and being laughed out of the arena, I have taken the side of the underdog, artificial sweeteners.

It puzzles me why some Fat Ugly people say they are concerned that artificial sweeteners may be dangerous. Many sugarholics consuming almost an IV bag of sugar a day worry about sweeteners. I am no scientist, doctor, or nutritionist, just a man who has survived through Vietnam, alcohol, drugs, smokes, and fat. Fat is much more scary than artificial sweeteners to me. Bring sweeteners on, and if your system is strong, you will probably not go down.

Since I was a kid, people told me sugar rots your teeth. They said it helps cause cavities. They told me sugar would make me hyperactive and higher than a helium balloon when combined with too much pop. They even had names for it, like "sugar buzz," "sugar jitters," or "sugar high."

Cowboys would call their girlfriends "Sugar." Calling girls "Sugar" did not cause cavities and usually got you a kiss, which was nice and calorie free. It might lead to marriage, but not fatness.

I see some of the biggest waddlers eating and drinking sugar-loaded drinks with domes of whipped cream, chocolate, and sprinkles. They should just get a garden hose loaded with sugar, put it in their mouths, and pull the trigger. Blow up five dress sizes with sugar sweets. Sugar seems like more than an innocent little thing in the sugar bowl.

Companies load cereal with sugar because sugar makes them taste better and you want more. They even make cereals sugar coated in case you are too tired or stupid to add your own sugar. Sugar is the key ingredient in many cereals, candy bars, doughnuts, and things that taste so good that you just must have one. Okay, must have 2, 3, 10, or more.

The Fat Warrior contends that the biggest sugar sabotage is honey. The health food freaks will have my head on this one. However, sugar-hidden calories embed in each honey drop. The calories hide in honey, which is disguised by the word "natural" and sold in health food stores. Honey sounds nice, and we call people honey with affection and love. Spread it on your peanut butter sandwich and call it a Snickers bar. Pour it in your tea and watch it grow on your bod. There are many carriers of calories for fat building, but none so well named as honey. **Well, now I have even made the bees mad.**

A song goes something like this: *Sugar in the morning, sugar in the evening, sugar at suppertime.* Artificial sweeteners have no songs written about them. Let's see, for possible titles:

- Loving You Makes Me Feel Splenda
- Kissing Your Feet Is Just Sweet'N Low
- You Are My Equal, Most of the Time
- NutraSweet Is So Sweet

I have been using Equal since it came out a long time ago, in a galaxy before Star Wars. I am normal, except for my writing and extra set of feet. I hope sugar hasn't decayed your sense of humor.

My son grew up without much sugar and in favor of artificial sweeteners. He is fine at the tender age of 30-ish and doing great. However, there was a time in his teens when I thought the Equal had his mind, but it turned out to be adolescence. This was a phase of immaturity shared by both father and son. He thought I was suffering from artificial sweetener insanity, and sometimes I was.

My point is that artificial sweeteners have been studied to death and have passed all the food and drug qualifications to be placed on the market as safe. I do not believe that if sugar came out today it could pass the same tests and classify as safe.

If I were a fattie and predisposing my bod to the added fatness provided by that calorie-laden sugar molecule, I would select Sweet'N Low. If I were heart-attack fat, everything else being equal, I would lose the sugar fatness and select the Equal. Selecting my tongue over my heart is not equal when it comes to life support machines.

Now, the only name that stands up to sugar is Splenda. Sugar is a cool name and memorialized in songs, poems, movies, and book titles. Even boxers and champions were called sugar, like Sugar Ray Leonard and Sugar Ray Robinson. Think of all the sugar names you know. I think Splenda has that kind of name appeal. Do you think a boxer's name one day will be Splenda?

Sugar is not addictive, but rather the taste is to die for! Unfortunately, too much sugar can make you fat, hyperactive, and unhealthy. In addition to causing tooth decay, sugar predisposes people to diseases like diabetes. People with diabetes have to test their blood sugar levels often. Have you ever heard of a NutraSweet monitor that was not a girlfriend? Have you ever heard of a doctor asking patients to watch their Splenda levels? We don't monitor Sweet'N Low for high or low levels. There are blood sugar tests, but not sweetener tests. Why is that?

Artificial sweeteners sure seem safer than sugar. I don't think a lot of people have been in the emergency room in a sweetener coma. I am not against sugar, but I do believe it pushes a lot more calories into fat bodies than ever suspected.

The point is, sugar can pump hundreds or thousands of calories per day into your bod. It hides in pop (Yankee "soda"), fruit drinks, ice cream, pies, brownies, cookies, muffins, candy, cereals, and other snacks and desserts. It is everywhere for you to wear its calories, so be sure to check the labels. If it lists sugar as one of the main ingredients, then skip that tasty thirst quencher or sweetened cereal and score points for BB. Be aware sugar also hides in your diet via sucrose, lactose, glucose, dextrose, honey, sorbitol, fructose, and maltose.

The Fat Warrior certainly understands the frustration of controlling your sweet tooth. A little sugar is okay and you will get it in your normal diet. However, too much sugar is hiding and secretly entering your bod in all forms of little taste treats. Add it up and the calories will kill you and your slimness.

Do the math: diet pop 0 calories, regular pop 110 calories. You do your thing, but I am always picking Splenda, Equal, NutraSweet, and

Sweet'N Low over calorie-laden sugar several times a day. See how many calories a day you can save by selecting artificial sweeteners. Keep your sweet tooth happy--select artificial sweeteners over sugar. Keep your body slimmer by selecting sweeteners as your winners.

The best thing may be to reduce both sugar and sweeteners from you bod. Healthy suggestions are to try adding in sensory appeal to your food with different tastes, textures, colors, and food temperatures. You'll be pleased as to what a difference this can make.

Confession: I Am a Sweetener Pimp

I felt somebody should stand up for artificial sweeteners because everybody wants to kick sugar in their faces. If you disagree, then I understand your fear of those little packets.

Okay, I will admit that I sound like a pimp for sweeteners and unfriendly to sugar. *My sweetest apologies.*

Notes

23

EATING OUT, NOT PIGGING OUT

The Chef Doesn't Discriminate-
She Makes the Menu for Fat or Fit

Date Plating

The first time Cutie and I went out for dinner, she decided once again that I was ready for a brave new venture to reduce my gut and make me movie-star handsome. I ordered my entree from the waiter--a New York strip steak, potato, and salad. Cutie told the waiter she would have the same thing.

Then the big surprise came. When the waiter asked her how she would like her steak done, she said she was having the same thing-- meaning what *I* ordered and we would split it. We would each like to have half, would they do that? "Certainly," he replied. They both forgot I was there and I lost my opportunity to say "Objection! Your Honor, I demand a no-share steak!"

I could not speak to stop this outrageous sharing, because it had removed my breath and speaking ability. I thought the maitre d' would murder us or have us imprisoned for dividing a steak in half, but apparently they are used to it and do it with a smile. They know they over-size the orders to satisfy the large appetite of the oinkers and make more money.

In Kansas where I grew up, we measured the quality of a steak by the size. Quantity *was* quality. At the Kansas Cowboys Steak House, they had a 48-ounce steak that completely hid the plate and the table. It was great quality and you got it free if you ate it all and lived. Some cowboys ate it all.

I have since gotten used to Cutie splitting our restaurant meals. It is now a changed lifestyle, and we have seen many other couples do it when dining with us. We know that if the other couple is BB, then they are more likely to split a meal. Hoggers only understand a banana split and clean their plates. One slim Cutie told me that she never cleans her plate and always leaves some for the Fat Fairy.

I think the first restaurant to start serving split portions should call it the Fat Warriors Date Plate. How fun to promote love and healthy bods!

__Share a Meal or Share a Date Plate:__ You can split one meal for two, even dessert. Share restaurant desserts or don't eat them at all. Many people don't want the huge plates of food, and that is how date plating evolved. Friday's Restaurants now serve smaller meals for less money.

Fataurants and Fat-Loading Equations

The number of times you eat out per week times 10 is the extra poundage you carry from Fataurants. Example: Eat out 4 times a week, multiplied by 10 equals 40 extra pounds that you wear from the Fataurants. Every 5 times you say "SuperSizeMyButt" adds 1 fat poundage unit. It is not just SuperSizing that adds pounds for you to wear and house, it is also the eating habits that you are developing eating out.

I must confess that I made up the multiples of eating out and fat pounds to get your attention. There are no statistics to prove the above, so just imagine what you think to be true. What you believe is true for you. Are you visualizing your new, leaner beautiful bod?

Value Meals Are Fat Deals

Do you want to get back at the parents who did not cook and took you to Fataurants for Value Meals? When you go to McDonald's or other fast food eateries and they order their SuperSizeMyButt combo heart attack with cholesterol artery-clogger shake, order a grilled chicken salad and diet drink. Sip your diet drink and ask them to tell you how their genetics or metabolism made them fat. Ask them what causes strokes, what causes diabetes, and how is it living the fat life? Right Size, not SuperSize.

> ***Electric Menu Board Rule:*** *If you order your meal from an electric menu board and receive it in less than three minutes, you are ordering fast fat food that should come with an exercise mat and personal trainer.*
>
> *Shovel it in, and then go to sleep on the exercise mat. Bring exercise mats for your Fat Ugly parents if they introduced you to Value Meal fat deals.*

Parents Are Either Role Models or Dough Models

It takes a lot of love to stand over the stove and prepare a healthy meal instead of driving to pork-up Fataurants. Don't tell me you do not have time to prepare a healthy meal for yourself or your family or you will observe my War Face and Combat Growl. Keep in mind that a healthy meal becomes calorie laden if it is swimming in cream sauces, buried in a pie crust, sautéed in butter, or has cheese toppings.

When you pork up your children at Fataurants, you are teaching them that Fuglies are good and bigger is better. The hamburger of today is almost two times the size of the hamburger in size and calories of 20 years ago. **The Unhappy Meal is actually a triple threat to a kid with a cheeseburger, fries, and sugar-laden Joke Coke. Be a Role Model, not a Dough Model. If you go to a Fataurant, skip the SuperSizeMyButt meal deal and go with a grilled chicken salad and Diet Coke or water instead.**

> *If you must order a SuperSizeMyButt meal deal, then split it with a friend. That way you'll only eat and wear half of it.*

Oink Up at All-You-Can-Eat Buffets (a/k/a "Stuffets")

When you see a sign that reads "All You Can Eat," then you should run from it at full speed! What they are really saying is, "For this amount of money we will let you shovel yourself until you bust. Come in and see if you can out-eat our profits." You can't. It is kind of like gambling in Las Vegas--you are going to lose money at all-you-can-eat stuffets, not pounds. You will enjoy the eating challenge and walk out feeling bloated and horrible.

Fat Warriors avoid the all-you-can-eat troughs. These are places where you eat like a pig and most patrons look like hoggers. Go inside and dare to stare and leave without eating. These are places where they actually charge you money for making decisions that might kill you or lose your ability to date Hot Bods. Pile your plate sky high and you can go back as many times as you can waddle. **It is the same as the Value Meal--*value your life and run*.** Never, ever eat at all-you-can-eat hog stuffets!

24

RELAPSE NEVER MEANS COLLAPSE

You do not have to win every inning. You just have to win the game.

Relapse, Not Collapse

Now that you feel motivated to eat better and get more exercise, remember that making positive lifestyle changes is challenging. You may even have tried lifestyle change programs previously, but without much success. Making lifestyle changes usually involves participating in a program more than once, as many people relapse.

The fact is that if you don't collapse and don't give up, but instead keep fighting you can't lose. When you quit you lose. **If you keep fighting, you will eventually realize that the emotional and physical pains of your food addictions prove to be the impetus to finally win your battle with them.**

One Plus Won Equals Three!

My two biggest win-then-fail battles are presented below for your enjoyment and my once torment: downsizing portions and night mousing. I would win only to fail, but renewed the fight with Right Size in sight. I wanted my Right Size so bad, I would not give up and would fight again.

I eventually won both battles, and picked up a bonus victory as a result. The pain and fat gain have long since disappeared. I won my battles one day at a time, with heavy casualties at times. However, victory is in my reduced belt buckle, flatter stomach, plus my bonus victory, and all permanently.

Right Sizing by Downsizing Portions

It was dueling banjos for me for both stomach stuffing and nighttime snacking. I failed many times before I got The 20-Minute Rule down for smaller portions. It took almost 90 days of winning and failing before The 20-Minute Rule and I became friends. Now I am happy with portion sizes that leave me satisfied and comfortable. I get up from the table feeling good about me instead of stuffed and bloated. I love life just a little bit better because of my Right-Sized portions and flatter stomach. I've also reduced my belt buckle by about two holes. I am not six pack abs, but my girth does not suggest birth anymore.

Props to you when you make this most important adjustment for your happiest, healthiest lifestyle. No reason to feel hungry, just eat Right-Sized portions for health and wealth of mind!

Night Mousing

Mousing is raiding the fridge in the middle of the night. This Fabit was associated with any wake-up call in the middle of the night. I became like Pavlov's dog, attacking the kitchen after dark. First it would be the fridge, then the pantry for potato chips, cookies, or both. Wow, that is a dream feast for nightmares.

Breaking the mousing habit was about a 60-day war between battle wins and losses. I just kept visualizing my flat stomach that would be mine, and sometime after 60 days the new lifestyle of not mousing was my victory. Now I am mouse free and proud of it because it affects my mind, body, sleep, and self-esteem. I am in control.

Add Your Bonus Victories

The added pleasure is that by winning my Right-Sized portions and late-night mousing battles, I also picked up a bonus victory for not eating after 7:30 p.m. Not eating after 7:30 p.m. is one of the most important battles to give you Right-Sizing victory and miles of smiles. The not eating after 7:30 p.m. victory is visible in my mirror every day. I am Looking Good, Feeling Good in my best Hot Bod, so turn up the music.

Remember, you don't win a war without losing some battles first.

Rethink Your Focus to NOT Be About WEIGHT LOSS

Nobody wants to lose weight. What people really want is to be their personal Right Size, which is more rewarding and permanent than just losing weight. Losing weight is nothing compared to having your best life possible. Think about it. Which is more valuable--a better life or losing weight for the short term? **Losing weight alone is worth a scuffle, but not a war. Having your best life complete with more joy, laughs, self-esteem, participation, health, and love life is worthy of war and fighting for every decision victory.** When you win that war, you will have lost your Fat Ugly and gained your Right Size for good.

If you lose weight, once you have accomplished that you get off the diet. Is the diet sustainable? If not, rebound upsizing occurs. The plan or diet has helped you accomplish the weight loss, but when the outside motivation ceases supporting you, you relapse back to fat.

So you put the weight right back on and you are perceived a failure and wallow in depression avoidance, when in fact you were a success. You lost the weight and achieved your weight goal. Take your before and after picture and know that you will be doing it again and again. **The problem is that losing weight was your goal and you crossed the finish line. You then had your after picture snapped along with your dreams.** If there is a before and after picture, beware of the camera angle. Their angle is the perpetual rebounding and getting you back because it increases their profits. It is the pay-up and pork-up cycle.

There should be no after picture because the camera can focus on weight gained and lost, but it cannot focus on decisions for a better life. You cannot take a picture of a decision or a better life. Or can you? **You must understand that it is not weight loss that should be your focus, but rather your best possible *life*. There is a huge difference.**

If You Stumble, Don't Give Up and You Will Win Your Race As Long As You Keep Running

You will hit setbacks and plateaus as you work to peel off the pounds. That is not defeat, but a part of the process needed to win lifestyle changes and the goal of a permanent better life. The winning battle strategy is to embrace these minor setbacks as a learning part of the process, an opportunity to muscle up your resolve and self-motivation. Learn and keep fighting to overcome Fugly decisions.

Picture how your life will be if you do not make lifestyle changes. Picture your life if you do. You will stall and fail, but you must get up and move forward. **Just keep your momentum going. You will be the life winner or loser, and you get to decide which.**

You will occasionally suffer from brain freeze and fail as a Fat Warrior. You only need to get up and keep deciding for more BBs.
Your reward is Body Beautiful,
having better health,
and better everything.

Yes everything.

25

FAT WARRIORS CHALLENGE NOW!

Take the Fat Warriors Challenge!

Waddler Watching Akin to Whale Watching

Know and observe how waddlers live and eat. That is what you *don't* want to do. Do you look like them? Do you eat like them? They probably do not exercise, or else they probably out-eat their exercise. Do you exercise? Do you out-eat your exercise? How do you think waddlers feel?

Watch what waddlers order at coffee shops, all-you-can-eat stuffets and fast food establishments. You will associate those things with waddlers and you may not order them. Embarrassment association factor: Watch what Fuglies order and you may not select the same thing when you make your ordering decisions.

McDonald's Challenge

McDonald's saw the Fat Warriors coming, so their math indicates. They added salads and subtracted trans fats. They have and are creating many healthy choices. Props to Mickey D's, the Fat Warriors salute your progress. You decide what gets loaded onto your spoon and fork, so fork up to your best interests at McD's.

McDonald's and other places have some excellent choices, just don't big out on the bad ones. Make BB menu choices. Show yourself, your friends, and family that you can make Body Beautiful decisions at many Fataurants. Make a game of it with your kids, **the Can-Do Challenge**. Your family can eat grilled chicken salads and watch the oinkers SuperSize themselves. These observations will have a dynamic impact on you and your kids. Observing what waddlers order will give you and your children insight to find the problem and answer in one word. It is not calories, foods, SuperSizeMyButt portions, or trans fats, but rather **decisions**. You can make BBs or Fuglies. It's your choice.

Take someone to lunch at McDonald's and order a healthy choice. Eat it while watching how the fatties eat and say, "That used to be me." You will feel great as you watch hippo hips order the SuperSizeMyButt fat baskets with cheeseburgers and fries while you are eating healthy.

Warriors stay away from SuperSizing their hips with their lips. Say NO to SuperSizeMyButt meals and YES to baked, broiled or grilled lean meat, fish, salads, soup, and whole grains. Set a sustainable goal for 10 Fuglies or less per month. A SuperSizeMyButt meal can be one, when you plan for it as one of your allowed 10 per month.

Do the Dare Stare!

Fat Warriors Dare: Start giving up your favorite treats and notice the difference between 10 minutes of taste fun and all day feeling great knowing you are not growing wide hide. Then you will understand the difference between minutes of taste and a lifetime of looking and feeling your best.

Is it a horror to Dare Stare and see being FU for the rest of your life? Fat lasts a lifetime if you don't throw yourself the lifeline of good decisions. The pleasure of BB decisions is measured by more fun and health. The pain of FU decisions is depression, bad looks, and bad health. Put that axiom on your spoon and lift to the mouth.

26

GIVE UP AND SHUT UP, OR FIGHT

Win Your Happiest, Healthiest Lifestyle

Only you can decide whether to give up or fight.

Fat Warriors Against Fat

We are at war against Fat Ugly and its effect on people. You are now beginning your war, and it will become your new, positive way of life. When you are Looking Good, Feeling Good, everything is more fun and life is beautiful. You are more attractive to the opposite sex, you are better in business, may make more money, and feel better around your children and significant other. You will be wearing happy smiles instead of Fugly frowns.

With Fat Warriors, there are no guarantees because we do not sell miracle pills or magic elixirs. **However, we do guarantee, and your judgment tells you, that if you make the right decisions you will win your war on fat and make your Right-Size goal a reality**.

We guarantee that Fat Warriors will be in your face and will war with you as our army helps you defeat Fat Ugly. We guarantee that you can put on your special War Face, give your Combat Growl, and start making BBs now!

It costs your body and your pocketbook to be Fat Ugly. Be hard on your fat and order it off your bod. Demand fat to leave you alone forever. Will it to leave, and then make the decisions to make it happen.

Life Is Too Short to Live It Fat Ugly

As you record in your ScoreBook, keep in mind that mastering this lifestyle change is an ongoing adventure. On the scales of life, you will lose fat pounds as you gain fat-fighting momentum and self-esteem. We congratulate you on taking this journey to become your personal Right Size. You now may join the Fat Warriors Nation.

Become a Fat Warriors Recruiter--recruit your friends, family, kids and grandchildren, and have fun fighting fat and making people happy!

27

PLEASE VISIT OUR WEBSITE AT
www.FatWarriorsNation.com

Fat Warriors Nation Needs Your Stories!

We need our readers to send us stories for future Fat Warriors books. Examples: **Fat Warriors Top Fat Ugly Stories** (what I did wrong, fat horror stories, this could happen to you stories, bad things that happen when you are fat stories, your top 10 Fabits, your top BB suggestions, etc.). Fat Warriors wants **100 ideas for lifestyle changes that make a positive difference**. We also need **100 fat failures**, as those stories are also highly impactful. **Send us your stories today, and they may end up in our books and seminars!**

Please share your **success stories and fat defeats** so that others may learn from your experiences. We appreciate your **experiences and advice to which parents and children can relate. Photos are welcome** only with your written permission to make public. We will not return photos or materials.

Your tips will help other people win their wars on Fat Ugly. Your stories and ideas will educate and inspire others, and may even save lives.

We also want **ideas for contests, challenges, tests, and attack fat war games, like Fattleship.** What games would you create and suggest? Be creative!

Your stories must be things that you want to share with the public and become the property of Fat Warriors, Inc. Send to **www.FatWarriorsNation.com**. If you wish to remain anonymous, do not sign your name. On the other hand, if you wish to sign your name and give permission to take your information into public venues, please supply your contact information. In both cases, we need your written permission to publish.

Fat Warriors welcome you to the Fat Warriors Nation. You will put on your War Face, and someday put the sunroof down and drive out in your new best Hot Bod!

Notes

Watch for Other Fat Warriors Books and Products at www.FatWarriorsNation.com

Books & e-books

Mind Matter Over Fatter Matter: How you can develop mind control to pilot your thoughts into you and your family's Best Bods and lifestyles. Expected release date July 2009.

Parents--Role Models or Dough Models: Helping parents with the positive role to raise Right Sized, healthy children, and avoid setting the example that will result in pain for fat children. Expected release date February 2010.

Eating Naked: The Fat Warriors guide to scrumptious eating based on recipes and meals stripped of their chemicals and additives. Projected release date to be announced.

Interact with the Fat Warriors Nation

Fat Warriors Boot Camps, Seminars, and Speeches: See our website at www.FatWarriorsNation.com.

Notes

FAT WARRIORS GLOSSARY

BB: Short for **B**ody **B**eautiful.

BB Average: Your Body Beautiful Average. To calculate your BB Average, take your total number of BB decisions and divide by your total number of BB and FU decisions.

BB Decisions: Decisions to eat **B**ody **B**eautiful foods that will help you attain your Best Bod permanently, like eating an apple instead of a piece of cake. A decision to exercise is a BB.

Big Out: Over-indulging in food.

Body Beautiful ("BB"): Your **B**ody **B**eautiful is a result of your **B**ody **B**eautiful decisions.

Cheat-Eating: Like cheating on your significant other, if you do it, you know it when you chew.

Cognitive Dissonance: The difference between the bod you have and the bod you want.

Combat Growl: You will earn and learn yours.

Date Plate: Splitting a restaurant meal between two people, even dessert.

Eating Naked: Strip chemicals, eat organic.

Fabit: A Fat Ugly habit, such as night snacking.

FantaSize: Positive visions of how and what you want your bod and lifestyle to be, such as a firmer bod, sexy flat stomach, and LGFG lifestyle.

Fat Bullies: Ice cream, sugar cereals, no exercise, pop, etc.

Fat Dome: Coffee house drinks with domes of whipped cream, chocolate, and other sugar-laden toppings.

Fat Tax: Tax that politicians would place on fat.

Fat Ugly ("FU"): The Ugly look of obesity. You know it when you see it and when you wear it.

Fat Warrior: What you will become by making decisions to attain your Best Bod. You will work your way up through the ranks. Join us, team up, and defeat fat!

Fataholic: Person who believes he or she is condemned to Fat Ugly because of an addiction to the taste pleasures of Fugly foods.

Fataurants: Fast food restaurants serving up tasty Fugly foods.

FatCorn: Popcorn laden with huge amounts of creamy butter.

FatCrap: Undesired additives and chemicals placed into processed foods. FatCrap is an ugly name for ugly chemicals.

Fatting Average: Your Fat Ugly Average. To calculate your Fatting Average, take your total number of FU decisions and divide by your total number of LG and FU decisions.

FU: Short for **Fat Ugly**.

FU Decision: A **Fat Ugly** decision that makes one fat, such as eating a brownie or TV-couching and crunching.

Fugly/Fuglies: Slang relating to Fat **Ugly** or **FU**.

Grabits: Grocery carts filled with Fabits are called Grabits.

Hogger: Another term for a Fat Ugly person. A waddler.

Hot Bod (body): Your best possible body that you will pay the price for and earn. This does not mean movie-star hot, but your realistic personal best body for looks and health.

Joke Coke: Sugar-laden soda that often accompanies a SuperSizeMyButt meal as if it is free, but comes with about 300 calories.

Law of Attraction: Theory that what you envision, think about, talk about, and associate with becomes reality in time. If you constantly think about Fat Ugly foods and weight gain, that will become your reality.

Law of Fattraction: Fat Warriors theory that if you think about fat, you will attract Fat Ugly.

LG: Short for Looking Good.

Looking Good, Feeling Good ("LGFG"): Lifestyle of self-esteem and joy when you are winning your war from FU to LG.

Mind Over Fatter: Using your mind to help you choose not to eat a Fugly.

MochaChocaLatte: Coffee drink loaded with tasty fat pleasures.

Mousing: Raiding the fridge in the middle of the night.

Pit-Bull Mentality: Total Can-Do attitude and determination to defeat fat. You will never give up because you have Pit-Bull mentality and are destined to win your war against Fat Ugly.

Pork Up: Gaining Fat Ugly.

Rebound Fat: Gaining Fat Ugly back, along with horrible depression plus the avoidance factor, after dieting.

Right Size/Right Sizing: Achieving the personal size and weight that is best for you.

Scale Tossing: Tossing scales in the trash or to a neighbor (at least into the closet for you to bring out once per month). Scale tossing can be fun when you toss a perfectly good scale to your neighbor. Then explain the Fat Warriors strategy behind scale tossing.

Scorebook/ScoreBooking: Keeping an ongoing record of LG and FU decisions. From this record you can calculate your BB Average and Fatting Average. ScoreBooking is the best way to tell if you are improving, winning or losing.

Self-Talk: What you say to yourself, composed by your thoughts, that may become your beliefs.

Stand-Snacking: Snacking or eating standing up.

Stuffet: Another word for an all-you-can-eat buffet restaurant.

SuperSizeMyButt: Ordering the economy-sized version of a Fat Ugly, calorie-laden meal of FU food, such as a huge cheeseburger, extra-large fries, and Joke Coke.

The 20-Minute Rule: Don't eat until stuffed. Instead, stop when comfortable, wait 20 minutes, and see if you still want more.

TV-ing: The art of eating and watching TV without awareness.

Waddler: Another term for a Fat Ugly person. A hogger.

War Face: Your personal determination mode to win your war against fat. The face you make to show that you are determined to stand your ground and fight Fat Ugly.

Weapons of Mass Ass Destruction (WMAD): Your brain, decisions, self-motivation, discipline, emotions, beliefs, accountability, and lifestyle changes form your arsenal against Fat Ugly.

YogaLight: Quick mental concentration for winning Right-Sizing decisions by visualizing.

FAT WARRIORS
RULES & LAWS

Electric Menu Board Rule: If you order your meal from an electric menu board and receive it in less than three minutes, you are ordering fast fat food that should come with an exercise mat and personal trainer.

Fat Warriors Law: The chances of winning your personal war on fat are directly proportional to your pain levels of owning Fat Ugly. The higher your pains of being fat, the higher your chances of defeating FU permanently. Understanding the embarrassment you feel, the scariness of facing health issues, and the thought of not being a good dating or mating prospect will help you fight back. The more these things hurt, the more they motivate you to fight and defeat. So put on your War Face, growl, and fight your Fuglies!

Fat Warriors Rule: Reduce your Fuglies to reduce your waistline.

Large Portion Rule: Eating large portions at any time makes the stomach full, but your brain may not get the message until 20 minutes later. This gives you time to stuff the stomach uncomfortably full. Loosen that belt, unbutton those jeans. If it curves out, then you will fill out. If you eat thin, the stomach stays in.

Law of Attraction: The Law of Attraction is a theory that what you envision, think about, talk about, and associate with becomes reality in time. It is like the movie "The Secret." What you visualize you will attract. Visualize healthy and you will attract healthy. Visualize driving your Best Bod and it will lead you to the Winner's Circle. Think about and visualize Looking Good, Feeling Good, and it will happen. Law of Attraction will help you battle fat.

Law of Dating Pool: Your dating pool is reduced in direct proportion to the amount of fat you've produced.

Law of Fattraction: Just as the Law of Attraction says that what you think about will come to you, if you are distracted from your goal by constantly thinking about the pleasures of Fugly foods you will attract Fat Ugly. This is the Fat Warriors Law of *Fattraction*. Visualize fat and you will attract fat.

Law of Forever Fat: The pleasure of temporary taste is stronger than my will to make good decisions. Therefore, I will wear the temporary fat pleasure and live with the fat lifestyle of depression, embarrassment, and bad health forever.

Law of Override Depression: Your body is the barometer of how you feel. If you look and feel Fat Ugly, that feeling will override to dominate your thoughts about yourself.

When you start Looking Good and Feeling Good (LGFG), that feeling will dominate your thoughts and beliefs. Your thoughts become your beliefs whether or not they are factual. What you believe you will achieve.

Law of Slow Is Faster: The amount of time it takes for you to take weight off quickly may be approximately the amount of time it will take you to gain it back. The slower it comes off, the longer it stays off. You are not in a hurry to Right Size. Your only focus is making decisions for permanent lifestyle changes.

Lost and Found Rule: I lost the fat, but fat found its way back in the same massive places.

Reversal of Taste Rule: Some good foods will not taste as good as fat foods at first, but the longer you eat healthy, the more you acquire a taste for healthy foods. The great news is that your taste buds will eventually lose their zest for the intense taste of fat foods.

Most good foods taste good and make you feel even better. Good foods promote health and happiness; bad foods promote high blood pressure, diabetes, low self-esteem, sad clothes, and other bad things. What is your choice for life?

Rule of Negative Decisions: When I make a negative decision, I feel bad. The more I make, the worse I feel.

Rule of Positive Decisions: When I make a positive decision, I feel good. The more I make, the better I feel.

Rule of Time & Taste: "If it tastes good, then I must have one or treat myself to one." In a matter of minutes, the good taste is gone, and the bad feelings linger, as does the fat forever. You wear and carry what you eat. For minutes fat foods taste real good, but make you feel bad for hours.

Small Plate Rule: Big Plate means more taste but added feelings of stuffiness. Small Plate means a comfortably full, flat stomach, and Body Beautiful pride. The flat stomach lasts. The enjoyment of a stuffed, fat stomach is over quickly and turns to sluggish depression. It is your choice. Go happy, go LG, go Right Size.

www.ingramcontent.com/pod-product-compliance
Lightning Source LLC
Chambersburg PA
CBHW070925270326
41927CB00011B/2721